D0787887

MAN-opause

MAN-opause

What Everyone Should Know about Treating Symptoms of Male Hormone Imbalance

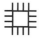

BRIAN R. CLEMENT
AND ANNA MARIA CLEMENT

ROWMAN & LITTLEFIELD
Lanham • Boulder • New York • London

Published by Rowman & Littlefield
An imprint of The Rowman & Littlefield Publishing Group, Inc.
4501 Forbes Boulevard, Suite 200, Lanham, Maryland 20706
www.rowman.com

6 Tinworth Street, London SE11 5AL, United Kingdom

British Library Cataloguing in Publication Information Available

Library of Congress Cataloging-in-Publication Data

Names: Clement, Brian R., 1951– author. | Clement, Anna Maria, author.
Title: Man-opause : what everyone should know about treating symptoms of male
     hormone imbalance / Brian R. Clement and Anna Maria Clement.
Description: Lanham : Rowman & Littlefield, [2020] | Includes bibliographical
     references and index. | Summary: "Everything a man—or woman—needs to
     know about the symptoms—irritability, depression, fatigue, weight gain—of
     male hormone imbalances can be found in this authoritative yet accessible book
     that reveals the latest science findings"— Provided by publisher.
Identifiers: LCCN 2019038356 (print) | LCCN 2019038357 (ebook) | ISBN
     9781538129340 (cloth ; alk. paper) | ISBN 9781538129357 (epub)
Subjects: LCSH: Climacteric, Male. | Middle-aged men—Health and hygiene.
Classification: LCC RC884 .C54 2020 (print) | LCC RC884 (ebook) | DDC
     616.6/93—dc23
LC record available at https://lccn.loc.gov/2019038356
LC ebook record available at https://lccn.loc.gov/2019038357

∞™ The paper used in this publication meets the minimum requirements of
American National Standard for Information Sciences—Permanence of Paper
for Printed Library Materials, ANSI/NISO Z39.48-1992.

CONTENTS

Introduction
Who in Your Life Has Irritable
Male Syndrome?

"If menopause is the silent passage, 'male menopause' is the unspeakable passage. It is fraught with secrecy, shame, and denial. It is much more fundamental than the ending of the fertile period of a woman's life, because it strikes at the core of what it is to be a man."

—GAIL SHEEHY, *UNDERSTANDING MEN'S PASSAGES*

SHORTLY AFTER THE BIRTH of their first child, when Rowan Pelling's husband turned fifty-one years old, his dark hair turned gray almost overnight. Soon afterward, she found him clutching his chest in horror one morning, muttering, "What on earth are these?"

What he had discovered was the appearance of flabby mounds of flesh on his chest, often snidely referred to as "man boobs." While these physical changes were disconcerting enough—for both of them—what really concerned her, more than anything, was the disturbing difference she saw in his personality.

"I'm not sure what's most galling about the mid-life 'change,'" Pelling wrote in Britain's *Telegraph* newspaper. "The mood swings, thickening midriff, saggy chest, aching joints, night sweats, memory loss, exhaustion, loss of libido, or general irascibility? Girl Guide's honor, I am genuinely curious about what symptom is the worst. But whenever I ask my husband, he bites my head off."[1]

Her husband was undergoing the sort of midlife hormonal changes that are the male equivalent of menopause symptoms experienced by women. While most men go through these sorts of changes, nothing this couple had ever read or heard could have prepared them for the jolting transformations and resulting relationship challenges that a progressive decline in male hormones triggers.

The clinical definition of this male life transition is *andropause*, a term first coined by medical specialists in 1967, referring to a progressive decline in male sex hormones, primarily testosterone, but also involving growth hormone and several others. At first, only a few symptoms were ascribed to this phenomenon, such as a loss of virility. With more medical research came the realization that men experience a wide range of hormonal decline symptoms, just as women do in menopause, and men experience these symptoms for far longer than is normally true for women.

Becoming a crotchety old man, irrespective of one's true biological age, was first identified as a hormonal failure in a 2001 study, published in a British reproductive science journal, in which the term *Irritable Male Syndrome* was used to describe the irritability, anxiety, and other confidence-sapping behavioral changes that are part of a cluster of male hormone decline symptoms.

"Is 'manopause' more widespread than we thought?" asked Rowan Pelling. She answered her own question by pointing out how "so many middle aged men feel so lost," as evidenced by their buying binges, whether it is flashy sports cars adorned with hood ornaments, young girlfriends, or "some form of male mood-altering contraband" from Amazon.

Whenever anyone asks this middle-aged andropause-rattled man how he is, Pelling said, "they had better be primed for a lengthy list of ailments (housemaid's knee, acid reflux, prostatitis, root canal work and athlete's foot) and the possibility he'll air his fear that his grandchildren will live in some form of post-catastrophe submerged, zombie-filled shopping mall by the year 2115."

European scientists did a review of the literature on andropause in 2015, finding evidence for "a distinct rise in the incidence of psychological disturbances among middle-aged men." The symptoms of emotional disorders documented in the science research, noted by the journal *Menopause Review*, included "moodiness, irritability, nervousness, depression, aggravation, fatigability, poor concentration, deteriorating memory, worse stress management and stress-related coping techniques, new aversion to certain activities that usually were enjoyable, or prolonged mood disorders."

As a result, andropausal men who "often have responsible professional functions and are at the peak of their careers" are experiencing health and psychological symptoms from hormonal declines that are "hindering their goals and result in overall [life] dissatisfaction."[2]

Are you concerned that your husband, your boyfriend, your father, or your son is fat, fatigued, grumpy, and dispirited, a candidate for Irritable Male Syndrome (or perhaps they are already a member in good standing)? If *you suspect the reason may be hormonal* and you have wondered what to do, this book was written with you in mind.

Healing the Male Fear of Gender Failure

For women, a cessation of menstruation marks the transition into menopause, whereas, for men, there is no clear biological signpost to mark the entry into andropause. Though both menopause and andropause involve a decline in hormones, it usually happens much more gradually with men and lasts longer, often decades and, for some men, even for the rest of their lives.

Because *andro* means male and *pause* means stopped, some men understandably react with revulsion and horror to any labeling insinuation that they have somehow "stopped" possessing what it takes to be a "real" man.

Since the medical establishment is predominantly male, to some extent, despite all of the scientific evidence, there exists an institutional denial about the existence of andropause—or at least a willful ignorance. It's a dismissive attitude that reinforces the denial many individual male patients feel when they are confronting dramatic life changes resulting from andropause symptoms.

"The only permission men of my generation have had to talk about something of this nature has been through taunting and teasing other men. Therefore, we could never acknowledge a 'weakness' of this sort without compromising our perceived manhood," observes

Dennis Marasco, a licensed professional counselor in Ohio who specializes in advising andropausal men.

"We men intuitively understand that as we age, things will change," continues Marasco. "But we assumed it would change gradually to the point that we wouldn't even notice it, or be aware of the impact on us, our actions or our relationships (including sexual relationships). We never thought that it would end up changing our perceptions of ourselves, which we have spent a lifetime developing."[3]

When a man's male identity is threatened, particularly his sexual identity, a first response is often to deny the existence of any problem. If that fails, a fallback position is to insist that "I can fix this by myself." If the man discovers he can't fix the andropause problem and its symptoms on his own, he may give up and resign himself to acceptance, declaring, "This is something I can't change, so I must learn to accept it."

None of these responses are healthy or helpful in improving a man's quality of life or the well-being of the people in his life who know and care about him. Dispelling this resistance, showing how and why the situation isn't hopeless, and proving that there are remedies for the host of symptoms are the reasons we decided to write this book.

We Offer Evidence-Based Natural Solutions

It didn't get much attention when it appeared in 2007, but it was nonetheless a revealing and important medical study. A group of randomly selected men from the Boston, Massachusetts, area—more than fifteen hundred of them—were medically observed over nearly two decades at the New England Research Institutes. Periodic blood tests measured their serum total testosterone and calculated their bioavailable testosterone.

"We observed a substantial age-independent decline in testosterone that does not appear to be attributable to health and lifestyle characteristics," wrote the research team in the *Journal of Clinical Endocrinology & Metabolism*. "The estimated population-level declines are greater in magnitude than the cross-sectional declines in testosterone typically associated with age."[4]

In other words, population-wide drops in testosterone levels (estimated at 22 percent between 1987 and 2004) are occurring far beyond what should have been predicted from this study, based on age-related differences in testosterone levels. (The age range of men in the study was forty-five to seventy-nine years.) What these findings portend, as implications for the long-term future of male fertility, hasn't even been contemplated yet.

How and why could this be happening?

The only explanation these study scientists could come up with is that "health or environmental effects" must be undermining male hormones and that scientific recognition of this phenomenon has been hidden from view in a growing mound of research data, erroneously attributed to normal male aging patterns that result in andropause.

A separate study by the same research team did find several confounding factors: with every four- to five-kilogram increase in a man's body mass index, or in the aftermath of losing a spouse, declines in total serum testosterone equaled the effects of about ten years of aging. That is a significant impact from just fat accumulation and feelings of grief.

In this book, we draw connections from environmental science studies showing the estrogenic (and testosterone-lowering) effects of many foods and personal care products and the role these endocrine disrupters are playing in the magnification of andropause symptoms. Among the solutions we offer, our suggestions of chemicals and products to avoid will go a long way toward helping readers create their own andropause mitigation and treatment plan.

Alongside a decline in testosterone during andropause, another key hormone diminishing with advancing age is human growth hormone (HGH), produced by the pituitary gland.

With falling HGH levels comes an array of musculoskeletal, metabolic, and cognitive conditions and other health issues. For example, you may experience reductions in your skeletal muscle and bone mass strength (your height will diminish as a result), and you may find fat accumulating around your waist, accompanied by a loss of virility, heightened cardiovascular risks, and a decline in mental acuity. All of these factors further compound the effects of testosterone depletion.

As with hormone replacement therapy for estrogen loss in women and testosterone loss in men, HGH replacement therapy has shown some positive effects; yet it remains a controversial approach because of medical concerns about its long-term safety, particularly regarding the risk of some cancers. We will evaluate all of the scientific evidence (pro and con) to enable readers to make their own informed decisions about the value of HGH therapy, as well as testosterone replacement therapy.

An alternative to HGH replacement that we consider comes from an entire body of plant-based science, using phytochemicals from various plants, to provide safe and effective treatments for a man's HGH loss. Phytochemicals are produced by plants as a defense against diseases and pests.

As an example, we will review science findings that identified three isoflavone phytochemicals—genistein, daidzein, and equol—as being particularly promising growth hormone supplement options. These nutrients are found in foods such as chickpeas and fava beans.

Supplementation with soy isoflavones is a cheap and easy way to begin addressing the wide spectrum of aging symptoms accompanying andropause, including HGH loss and its related health complications. Married to this approach are lifestyle changes, including a healthy diet coupled with resistance exercise training, which we also explain in detail, based on the latest science findings, in order for readers to create their own age-management plan for life.

Creating a personal treatment plan for the symptoms of andropause needs to be holistic, embracing dietary changes, an exercise program, stress management, hormone balancing, and much more. It's a comprehensive lifestyle approach that draws upon the latest evidence-based solutions.

When Menopause Mates with Andropause

As the authors of this book, we are a couple who have gone through our andropause and menopause years together. The symptoms we experienced were almost nonexistent, compared to other people our age, thanks to the lifelong health and dietary practices we have followed and describe in these pages.

As you will find in the last chapter of this book, if you are a man and woman in a dating relationship, or you are married and find yourselves experiencing hormone imbalances simultaneously, there may be relationship consequences you never could have imagined. The same is also true for andropausal men in relationship with men. If they are all going through hormonal changes together, the mental and physical health challenges remain similar.

When menopause occurs at the same time as andropause, which we see regularly in our visitors at the Hippocrates Health Institute, it becomes what two endocrinologists a few years ago called "couplepause"—a shared experience resulting in the potential for relationship disharmony, particularly from sexual dysfunction and misunderstandings surrounding that experience.

Some couples may be going through andropause and menopause simultaneously and enduring these changes while their children are also going through adolescence. All of these hormonal imbalances occurring together, affecting all members of a family at once, can become a recipe for conflict, turning home life into a virtual emotional war zone.

Symptoms of menopause in women, such as hot flashes, mood changes, and loss of libido, when coupled with symptoms of andropause in men, characterized by irritability, fatigue, and loss of sexual function (and yes, even hot flashes), can make it seem like a relationship is deteriorating, especially if the underlying hormonal declines are left untreated. This may be one contributing factor to the greater incidence of divorce occurring after grown children leave home.

If one partner in the relationship gets treated with hormone replacement therapy and the other doesn't, the untreated partner can actually experience a range of heightened psychological impacts, such as depression. If one partner regains his or her libido while the other doesn't, that situation could provide the seeds for temptation and philandering. If both partners undertake treatment together, as this book recommends, the odds of treatment success and a higher quality of life for both spouses go up exponentially.

By educating and treating both partners simultaneously (as we will describe how to do in this book), the impacts of midlife hormonal declines can be mitigated with a mutual support system to enhance treatment effectiveness. Until now, no book has revealed this "couplepause" condition or offered advice to couples on how to deal with the symptoms of this underpublicized and little understood subject.

If you are a man, you no longer need to suffer (and, as a result, be insufferable to others) while experiencing the Irritable Male Syndrome effects of andropause. If you are a woman, you no longer need to feel helpless in your desire to help the men in your life, as declining hormones impact their health and test their relationship with you and others, while undermining their overall quality of life.

MAN-opause (as we call it) is a treatable collection of symptoms. It is also a manageable and sometimes preventable condition and we will show you how to do just that.

That cluster of midlife hormonal declines called andropause can be a significant life challenge, one that nearly all men will eventually face; yet very few of them even realize the condition exists, much less that the vexing symptoms they are experiencing can be remedied.

Ask any dozen men or women whether they are aware that men go through an entire set of symptoms of hormonal imbalance, similar to what most women endure with menopause, and you will probably be met with blank stares or incredulity.

Using the latest medical science findings, *MAN-opause* explains in understandable language how any man—with or without a woman's participation—can take proactive steps, at any stage of life, to neutralize the impact of andropause and its wide range of debilitating symptoms.

We urge you to treat this book as a sort of owner's education manual for men and also for the women in their life, since it is often the women who inspire and coax men to break through self-imposed layers of denial in order to seek help when they are encountering health challenges.

Give Yourself This Andropause Assessment
Which Symptoms Describe You . . . or the Men in Your Life?

Bone Brittleness: When bone fractures occur more easily and you are experiencing chronic bone and joint weakness, it may be due to low testosterone levels. This condition could lead to complications, such as osteoporosis.

Brain "Fog": No longer feeling mental sharpness and displaying memory lapses unrelated to early-onset Alzheimer's. Fuzziness in thinking may be a result of low testosterone experienced during andropause.

Breast Growth: A man notices he is growing breasts and having larger breasts is "not his thing." This chest flab from weight gain may be a consequence of the low testosterone production from the andropause process of aging.

Fatigue: Being tired all the time, no matter how much caffeine is ingested, may signal low testosterone caused by andropause. As low testosterone affects sleep quality, lethargy and tiredness can be intensified.

Hair Thinning: A lowering of a man's testosterone production, beginning about forty years of age, can produce hair loss that has a visible impact on the head, chest, legs, and under the arms and even in the thickness of pubic hair.

Mood Changes: If a man becomes irritable for no apparent reason, or releases anger at the slightest provocation, or

develops depressive moods, he may be suffering from the
hormonal imbalances caused by age-triggered andropause.

Muscle Mass Deteriorates: An average man's lean body mass
decreases by about 10 percent every decade due to aging and
lower testosterone production. As a man loses muscle mass,
he gains even more body fat.

Prostate Enlarges: Andropause contributes to prostate
enlargement, which in turn produces increased frequency
to urinate, particularly at night. Other urinary symptoms
appear, such as incontinence.

Sexual Dysfunction: A man whose testosterone levels are
declining no longer wakes up in the morning with an
erection. He will also find that erections take longer to
obtain and he no longer feels a frequency of sexual desire.
A man's penis and scrotum may also undergo shrinkage
from testosterone deprivation.

Sleep Quality Declines: Insomnia can be due to low
testosterone. Because growth hormone is produced during
sleep, disturbances of natural sleep rhythms can deplete
this hormone, adding to the impact already being caused
by andropause.

Stress Overwhelms: Hormone levels are affected by sleep
quality and chronic stress. One condition reinforces the
other. A chronic release of cortisol, the stress hormone,
undermines testosterone levels.

Weight Gain/Obesity: As a man puts on extra pounds, his
testosterone is converted into estrogen. That further reduces
his testicles' ability to produce more testosterone. This cycle
is further exacerbated by andropause having the effect of
lowering testosterone, producing even more fat retention.

A Short Symptom Assessment Quiz

This questionnaire, used by medical specialists to identify and gauge
the severity of andropause symptoms, is called the Androgen Deficiency in Aging Males (ADAM) scale.

Here are the ten questions used in the assessment scale.

1. Do you have a decrease in libido or sex drive?
2. Do you have a lack of energy?
3. Do you have a decrease in strength and/or endurance?
4. Have you lost height?
5. Have you noticed a decrease in your enjoyment of life?
6. Do you feel sad and/or grumpy?
7. Are your erections less strong?
8. Have you noticed a recent deterioration in your ability to exercise?
9. Do you fall asleep after dinner?
10. Has there been a recent deterioration in your performance at work?

If you answer yes to questions 1 or 7, or yes to three or more of the other questions, you might be diagnosable as having andropause.

If your levels are found to be below the norm (total testosterone of below 300 ng/dL, or free testosterone below 5 ng/dL), and you answered yes to four or more of the questions, you may be diagnosed as being in andropause. It is also possible that you could have low testosterone even though you don't yet show evidence for some, or most, of the symptoms of andropause.[1]

Why You Should Trust This Assessment Scale

Numerous science studies have been conducted testing the reliability of the Saint Louis University Androgen Deficiency in the Aging Male (ADAM) assessment scale questionnaire, which was first developed in 2000, by a team of researchers who published it in the journal *Metabolism*.[2]

As an example, in 2010, a team of urologists from three U.S. and Canadian universities gave the ADAM questionnaire to thirty-four men with an average age of sixty-two years, who also then had their testosterone levels measured. A "statistically significant correlation" was found between the questionnaire results and the testosterone results. One-third of the men had serum testosterone levels below 300 ng/mL, qualifying them as hypogonadal, meaning that their testicles don't produce healthy levels of testosterone and sperm.[3]

To determine whether the ADAM questionnaire is also effective in assessing testosterone deficiencies among Chinese men, it was given to 176 men, average age of fifty-four years, who were patients in a psychiatric clinic suffering from anxiety or depression.

A remarkable 93 percent of them were found to be experiencing an impairment of life quality based on having affirmative responses to the ADAM questions about sexual functioning. Though there can be some debate about whether being anxious and/or depressed caused their failure of sexual functioning, finding low testosterone seemed to indicate a connection between the symptoms of andropause and their sexual and psychological states of well-being.[4]

How Widespread Is Andropause and Low Testosterone?

One of the largest community-based screening programs ever undertaken involved 5,071 men in Colorado who took health questionnaires and had their testosterone levels tested and compared, in 2014, by a team of university urologists.

Among the findings, published in the *Journal of Men's Health*, were:

- The average testosterone level was 378.6 ng/dL.
- Nearly half of the men had testosterone deficiency.
- Men who exercised five times or more per week had levels of 391, compared with 360 for men exercising less or not at all.
- Men who were overweight by thirty pounds or more had scores averaging 293, compared to 421 if they had normal weight.
- For those with adult-onset diabetes who were also overweight, their risk for testosterone deficiency increased from 49 percent to 62 percent.[5]

Some Key Terminology to Keep in Mind

The following terms relate to andropause and its symptoms and are used throughout this book:

Andropause: A constellation of brain and body symptoms marking a male's passage into hormonal decline, as a result of a combination of lifestyle and aging; also referred to in medical circles as testosterone deficiency syndrome, or androgen deficiency of the aging male. Still another term for this condition is *male menopause*, which was first medically identified in 1944, in a study by two physicians, published in the *Journal of the American Medical Association*, in which the symptoms were described as a "deteriorated general and sexual condition in men."

Hypogonadism: A medical term for when testosterone levels fall below 300 ng/dL, as a result of a physical abnormality in the testes or brain; as contrasted with andropause, which is considered by the medical establishment to be a "natural" hormonal decline with age.

Testosterone: Called the primary male sex hormone, it's produced by the testes and regulated by the pituitary gland and the hypothalamus brain region. Beginning around age thirty, testosterone levels drop by 1–2 percent a year until, by age eighty, most men will have levels below what they possessed when they entered puberty. Women also produce testosterone, at small levels in their ovaries, but their levels are far lower than men's and they also decline with age.

Estrogen: Known as the female sex hormone, men also produce tiny amounts of it through an enzyme called aromatase, which transforms estrogen into estradiol, which in turn, helps modulate male libido and erectile function. Men need estrogen, as women do, just not in excessive amounts. It's important for intimacy, receptivity, and touching. Too little of it may result in heart disease. Too much of it actually lowers the amount of testosterone in the body, hastening the symptoms of andropause. Among the triggers for excess estrogen in the male body: too much body fat, too little zinc and vitamin C, too much alcohol, cholesterol fighting medications, and exposure to synthetic chemicals that are xenoestrogens (mimics of estrogen).

Growth Hormone (GH): Made by the pituitary gland, it controls growth and metabolism, and it increases muscle mass while decreasing body fat. Called a peptide hormone, it stimulates cell growth and regeneration. Humans experience a steady decline in growth hormone beginning with middle age. HGH (human growth hormone) is a controversial replacement therapy for growth hormone deficiency, administered as an injection under the skin, to treat diminishing bone and muscle mass and other age-related body changes.

DHEA (dehydroespiandrosterone): An androgen hormone produced by the adrenal glands; it's important (as a precursor) to testosterone production, and like testosterone, DHEA declines with age. Saliva tests are most effective in measuring DHEA levels. When the body is stressed, it secretes DHEA, along with cortisol, as a sort of counterbalance in order to calm emotions, act as a stress manager, and improve memory.

DHT (dihydrotestosterone): During embryo development, it causes the formation of the penis, scrotum, and prostate; later in life it's a metabolite of testosterone (meaning transformed into, as it is broken down) and plays a role in prostate growth and male balding.

Insulin-Like Growth Factor 1 (IGF-1): Several peptide hormones, found naturally in the blood, that stimulate cell growth and help to build muscle by regulating the effects of growth hormone. Their levels decrease with age.

Luteinizing Hormone (LH): Released by the pituitary gland, it travels through the bloodstream to the testes, where it helps to control the release of testosterone.

Sex Hormone–Binding Globulin (SHBG): A protein made in the liver that binds to estrogen, DHT, and testosterone. It controls the amount of testosterone the male body can use. Age as well as obesity and type 2 diabetes can lower SHBG levels.

Untreated Andropause Undermines Male Health

2

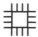

O NE OF OUR ASSOCIATES did an informal survey to help us determine how far in the shadows public knowledge of andropause and the impact of male hormone decline reaches into our culture. Randall Fitzgerald conducted his informal survey by randomly asking numerous men in their fifties and sixties, "Have you entered andropause yet?"

What he uniformly got in response were puzzled expressions or lame attempts at jokes or wisecracks. All of the men had heard of testosterone, but when he explained how low testosterone was only part of a larger health challenge, a single spoke (albeit an important one) in a wheel of hormonal changes that occur with age and resemble the symptoms of menopause in women, the men he spoke to were incredulous.

One of those surveyed even voiced the opinion that the condition was fake medical news. "Why haven't I ever heard about this condition before?" the doubter demanded. "If this really existed, wouldn't my doctor have warned me?"

Next, Fitzgerald tried the question out on a group of his wife's female friends. They had never heard the word *andropause* or the conditions it described, either, but when he detailed some of the classic symptoms, including irritability, fatigue, sleeplessness, waistline fat retention, and a loss of virility, it was as if a collective light bulb of recognition clicked on. There was knowing laughter followed by curiosity and a lot of questions.

These women knew intuitively the condition existed, even if they had never heard the terminology describing it before, because they were seeing firsthand the hormonal symptoms exhibited among the men in their lives. They were seeing it not just among husbands or boyfriends but also among their sons, fathers, brothers, and male coworkers.

"So maybe that's why my husband recently gained a lot of weight and became so short-tempered," one woman remarked. Said another, "That could explain why my boyfriend lost interest in sex."

Going back to the earlier question the doubter raised, *why are* most physicians either unaware of andropause or else so indifferent to its symptoms and the suffering this condition causes that they don't bother to educate their patients?

It may simply be that most traditional medicine physicians never received medical school training enabling them to recognize the symptoms of andropause. On top of that, many physicians simply don't have the time to read or translate what they read in the medical literature and integrate that into their practice. Others may be close minded or suspicious of natural hormone replacement treatments for low testosterone and andropause.

When a man comes to a physician complaining of depression, for example, the physician will usually prescribe an antidepressant, rather than check for low testosterone, which can also be a trigger for depression. Most physicians simply don't know to check for a link between mood changes and hormone levels.

Given that situation, how can we expect most consumers of health care to even know to ask questions about the impact of their hormones on their brain or their body? That lack of authoritative support from caregivers places a lot more pressure and responsibility on patients to do their own research exploring treatment options.

Are Midlife Crises Related to Andropause?

Dr. Lawrence Komer, who treats andropause patients in Canada, described the case of a fifty-two-year-old patient of his, named Roy, an electronics firm executive, who "has not been himself lately." Roy's relationship with his wife is strained, they often argue, and it has been weeks since they were last sexual with each other. Roy feels tired much of the time, has lost his drive to excel, and his co-workers have also noticed that "he is edgy and often unreasonable in his demands."

An outside observer might surmise that Roy is showing the symptoms of having a midlife crisis, though Roy chalked it all up to "I must be getting old." Dr. Komer, based on decades of experience treating the condition, came to a different conclusion. Roy shows all the symptoms of entering andropause.[1]

It's certainly understandable to wonder whether there is a clear difference between male menopause and a male midlife crisis. After all, we've all heard about men who, on entering their forties or fifties, suddenly want to act like teenagers again and abandon their family responsibilities to spend money on flashy new sports cars and having affairs behind their wife's back.

We don't know of any science studies that have measured the testosterone levels of these men going through a second childhood, though we wouldn't be surprised if testing revealed that they, too, were entering andropause. Instead of being irritable males, they act out the hormonal change by being irresponsible males.

Other men have been characterized as being in the throes of a midlife crisis simply by being morose, filled with self-doubt, or even feeling chronically depressed about the choices they have made in life and the regrets they feel about their life's direction.

Again, we don't know of any clinical studies being done on their hormone levels, but we wouldn't be surprised if a connection was found, particularly since moodiness and depression have been labeled as classic symptoms of low testosterone and andropause.

"Some women who live with a husband with Irritable Male Syndrome feel they are to blame for their husband's erratic behavior, short temper, and grumpy attitude. Ladies, it's not your fault," observed Tom Nikkola, a Minnesota wellness coach who has counseled men in andropause.[2]

Nikkola asks his clients a series of questions to help them determine whether they are an irritable male (or a midlife-crisis male) as a result of low testosterone. Do any of the following sound like you or someone you know?

- "You're a ticking time bomb. Sometimes you're kind, considerate, and selfless. Other times you are a selfish jerk. You're especially poopy toward those you love the most."
- "You feel depressed. Nothing excites you or motivates you. You don't feel like you have any 'fight' left in you. Even the stuff you used to stand up for, you'd prefer to ignore."
- "Your body feels more fragile and looks flabbier. You've gotten weak and soft. You don't need to shave as often, and your moobs (yeah, man boobs), where did those come from?"
- "The only thing that excites you in the bedroom is going to sleep, and you can't remember the last time you woke up with an erection . . . come to think of it, you can't remember a lot of things."

For a lot of men, says Nikkola, this has become their normal, real life, and "most guys don't say or do anything about it because if they did, they'd have to admit something is wrong."

Men Have Hormonal Cycles, Too

Biologist Dr. Winifred Cutler, an expert on hormonal cycles who has published dozens of scientific papers on the subject, points out how men have a hormonal rhythm, just as women do. A man's cycle might last a few minutes a day, or be seasonal, or even last a lifetime. For example, during sleep the testosterone levels rise each hour until morning, when at their peak, bringing the so-called "morning erections." Levels reach their lowest in the late afternoon.

In her book, *Love Cycles: The Science of Intimacy*, Dr. Cutler called these rhythms "the hormonal symphony of men." Hormonal secretions, according to Cutler, reach their peak in men during October (16 percent higher) and their lowest levels occur in April (22 percent lower). Though men have monthly hormonal cycles, just as women do, men's cycles are more unpredictable.[3]

We do see evidence of these daily and monthly fluctuations influencing the male temperament—producing testiness, irritability, and control issues—all far more frequently than most men would like to admit. This pattern contributes to the Irritable Male Syndrome that afflicts men as their testosterone levels decline with age.

"Hormonal cycles? That sounds too 'fem' for many of us to even contemplate," wrote psychotherapist Jed Diamond, in a 2012 article for GoodTherapy.org. "I first began to recognize that there might be more going on inside me when I began doing research on andropause, or male menopause, in the early 1990s. I was seeing changes going on with midlife men at my health clinic that seemed similar to what I saw with women going through menopause. Many of the men were having 'night sweats' and 'hot flashes.' Others were on an emotional rollercoaster, up one minute and down the next."[4]

Diamond began interviewing men in midlife, as well as women, to find out what they were seeing and experiencing. "Most of the men thought the idea that they were 'hormonal' was ridiculous. Most of the women had a different view. 'Well, it's about time you guys finally figured out you're hormonal,'" a wife told Diamond.

Women have historically been ridiculed, disparaged, shamed, or dismissed out of hand, particularly in workplaces, for being "hormonal" when they evidence any signs of the mood swings associated with menstruation or menopause. This "hormonal woman" stigma has been historically used to reinforce stereotypes and give men excuses to relegate women to lower rungs of the salary and advancement ladders.

We must wonder whether turnabout will be fair play, once andropause becomes better known, acknowledged, and accepted as a male hormonal phenomenon. Will men also have to bear these indignities of a stigma surrounding their moodiness and irritability?

Some Andropausal Men Experience Hot Flashes, Too

Most women undergoing menopause know them all too well— sudden feelings of their body being on fire, the sensation of hot flashing, and the sleep-disturbing night sweats accompanying them. It's not a gender-specific experience, despite the fact it is underpublicized in men because of a blanket of denial men have thrown over it.

Many men in the throes of andropause also have hot flashes and night sweats, as a result of testosterone deficiency, though the phenomenon in them is both underreported and understudied. The most direct research has been done on prostate cancer patients using androgen (testosterone) deprivation therapy as part of their treatment.

One such study, done at the Institute of Psychiatry at King's College London, evaluated the frequency and intensity of hot flashes and night sweats in a group of men after they received androgen-deprivation therapy and uncovered a pattern of reactions among them showing a fear of their manhood being under attack.[5] The study authors reported that "there were men who held beliefs about the impact of flashes on their perceptions of traditional gender roles, who experienced shame and embarrassment due to concerns about the perceptions by others and who experienced feelings of powerlessness over flashes." These reactions were based on their upbringing, and though the actual experiences of hot flashing and night sweats were physically similar to what women in menopause encounter, they "differed in terms of the influence of masculinity beliefs."

So, there we have another clue to the origins and nature of the Irritable Male Syndrome. These men feel powerless over their condition. It scares them; their macho denial defenses are crumbling in the face of it, and so they retreat into numbed silence or verbally lash out at everyone around them. Because the medical establishment remains predominantly male, there also exists an institutional denial about the existence of andropause, a dismissive attitude that magnifies the denial individual male patients feel when faced with dramatic life changes resulting from andropause and its symptoms.

When a man's male identity is threatened (particularly his sexual identity), if his first response of denying the existence of the problem fails, a fallback position is often to insist that "I can fix this by myself." If the man ultimately finds he can't fix the andropause problem on his own, he may give up and resign himself to acceptance, declaring, "I must learn to accept it."

None of those approaches is healthy, especially because, as you will find out in later chapters of this book, natural remedies exist that can give men back their sense of being empowered to help themselves.

Andropause Can Both Cause and Intensify Anxiety and Depression

There is a "chicken or egg" type of quandary with many of the symptoms of andropause. Does low testosterone cause the symptoms, or do the symptoms cause or exacerbate low testosterone and andropause? In many cases, cause and effect are a feedback loop, inextricably intertwined.

An example is the quandary surrounding the question of depression and its impact on sexual functioning. A study assessment of psychiatric hospital outpatients was designed to distinguish whether low testosterone, or anxiety and depression, had more of a negative effect on sexuality.

Researchers determined that impaired sexual potency wasn't significantly associated with anxiety or depression, but anxiety and depression do make many of the classic symptoms of aging, leading to sexual dysfunction, more severe. The results, published in the journal *Clinical Interventions in Aging*, concluded that "impaired sexual potency should raise the suspicion of androgen (testosterone) deficiency, rather than depression and anxiety, among middle-aged or older male psychiatric outpatients."[6]

Get to Know What "T" Does to You and for You

It's important to know and measure the difference between a man's free testosterone levels (normal range 25–30 picograms per milliliter) and his total testosterone (normal range 400–600 ng/dL). Quick definition: Total T is all of the testosterone in your system when measured, including T that is "bound" to sex hormone–binding globulin, or to albumin; by contrast, free T is unbound and circulates more widely.

A good analogy for the important difference between free T and total T was provided by the website Prostate.net: *"The difference between 'bio-available' T and 'total' T is a bit like the difference between body fat percentage and total weight. You might weigh a healthy sounding 180 pounds, but if 33 percent of that is body fat, you're definitely less than healthy."*

Research by a British andropause expert Dr. Malcolm Carruthers determined that men with symptoms of andropause usually had low levels of free testosterone (75 percent of them), whereas only about 13 percent of the men he surveyed registered low levels of total testosterone. That meant the total testosterone measures could result in andropause going undiagnosed.

In 1939, testosterone was first synthesized in a laboratory and, in the decades since, two versions emerged for use as a replacement therapy in men: synthetic and bioidentical. Though bioidentical isn't the same as "natural," the term *bioidentical* means its chemical structure is just like the structure of the testosterone the male body produces. By contrast, synthetic testosterone has been modified in its structure to aid in absorption by the body, which can make it more prone to adverse side effects compared to bioidentical.

Ways for men to take bioidentical or synthetic testosterones include skin injections, skin creams, gels, and a skin patch with pellets, or it can be taken orally. (More on all of this, including the relative effectiveness and safety of each form of administration, can be found in chapter 17.)

Note Racial/Ethnic Differences in Measuring Testosterone Levels

To help determine whether testosterone and related hormone levels account for why black men have higher prostate cancer rates than white or Hispanic men, teams of scientists have conducted widespread blood testing among those ethnic groups, with interesting results.

German cancer researchers, in 2007, tested 1,413 men—white, non-Hispanic blacks, and Mexican Americans—and compared their serum testosterone, estradiol, and SHBG (sex hormone–binding globulin) concentrations, after adjusting for their age, body fat percentage, alcohol and smoking use, and physical activity.

It was found that testosterone levels were higher in Mexican Americans than either whites or blacks, whereas non-Hispanic blacks had higher estradiol concentrations. These findings prompted the research team to urge that estradiol, along with testosterone, be used as measures of possible prostate cancer risk.

In 2013, scientists at the Johns Hopkins Bloomberg School of Public Health measured serum testosterone, estradiol, and SHBG levels in 134 males, aged twelve to nineteen years. They found that these Mexican American adolescent males had a higher testosterone concentration than whites and blacks, whereas white males had higher levels of estradiol than blacks and Mexican Americans.

A third study, in 2015, by University of Florida scientists, tested 355 black and 631 white males. They ranged in age from twelve to thirty-nine years. Between the ages of twelve and fifteen, black males had lower testosterone levels than white males. But these levels increased rapidly with age "and reached higher and earlier peak levels in black males compared to white males at twenty to thirty years of age. After reaching a peak level, testosterone levels declined earlier in black males than in white. Further analyses showed that black males had considerably higher levels of testosterone compared to white males aged twenty to thirty-nine years."

These scientists concluded their study results, in showing the faster decrease in testosterone levels among blacks, with increasing age, may account for racial disparities seen in prostate cancer rates. "Our findings also suggest that personalized medication for hormone replacement therapy may be necessary to avoid sudden drops in testosterone levels, particularly for black males."[7, 8, 9]

How Andropause Creates Health Challenges

As if you already didn't have enough age-related challenges in life that you thought you had to grapple with, a drop in your testosterone heralds the onset of that broader health condition, andropause, with its full range of debilitating symptoms.

From about the age of forty years on, all of the major male hormones, most particularly testosterone, start a steady decline in production levels, resulting in that constellation of physical and psychological symptoms known as andropause (clinically, it's known as androgen deficiency of the aging male, or late-onset hypogonadism).

It's a period in life during which many men feel a "midlife crisis," or what's called the "senior slump," sometimes nicknamed "male menopause."

For women, the cessation of menstruation marks the transition into menopause, whereas for men, there is no clear biological signpost to mark the entry into andropause. Though both menopause and andropause involve a decline in hormones, for women, most who go through it may be affected for just a few years in their fifties. With men, hormonal degradation usually happens much more gradually and lasts longer, often decades, even a lifetime.

Because andropause occurs over decades and persists, *most men will feel the effects in profound, life-changing ways.*

This is now even truer than ever, because testosterone loss is apparently being accelerated by environmental factors, one trigger possibility being the hormone-disrupting synthetic chemicals found in personal care products and the testosterone-depleting estrogens showing up in some processed foods.

In many respects, the range of symptoms seen and felt by men age forty and beyond resembles their entry into a second childhood. Andropause renders their sexual functions to almost pre-puberty, as their penis and scrotum shrink, erections fade away, and sexual desire diminishes. Some men are left with nothing more than memories of having had a sexually active past.

It's important to keep in mind that though testosterone is the hormone with the most impactful age-related decline—about 10 to 15 percent in drops per decade for the average male—other declining hormones also play a role in creating the constellation of symptoms of andropause: these include growth hormone, thyroxine, and DHEA.

Even as men's testosterone levels are declining, their estrogen hormones are increasing, by as much as 50 percent, and that, in turn, helps the prostate gland to enlarge and trigger benign prostatic hyperplasia (BPH). As anyone who has had it can attest, BPH restricts the urethra, resulting in urinary symptoms.

As a man gains weight, particularly in his midsection, having more fat means testosterone is more quickly converted to estrogen. That negative cycle further magnifies if the man is exposed to more estrogen hiding in his personal care products and from what he consumes out of our food supply.

As bioavailable testosterone levels drop 10 percent every decade, sex hormone–binding globulin (SHBG) increases, which is important because SHBG traps circulating testosterone until much

of it is no longer bioavailable to the body's needs. It's a reinforc-
ing cycle.

Early-onset andropause can also be triggered by other factors:
chronic stress, chronic negativity and toxic attitudes, rapid obesity,
and the interactions of medications with hormone-altering side effects.

You don't need a road map of all these cascading symptoms laid
out in front of you to sense how life changing this entire pattern can
be for any man.

"I suspect that we'd all be better off if we recognize that men,
like women, have our own challenges dealing with our hormones,"
writes psychotherapist Jed Diamond. "Knowing and accepting our
hormonal cycles may be the most important knowing we can have
about what it means to be a man."

Diseases and Health Conditions Connected to Low Testosterone

Titled "The Dark Side of Testosterone Deficiency," a series of study
reviews published in the *Journal of Andrology* in 2009 laid out an overview of the known science, showing how this deficiency, at any age,
is a risk factor for a range of diseases, most particularly, cardiovascular
disease and type 2 diabetes.

"A considerable body of evidence exists suggesting that androgen
deficiency contributes to the onset, progression, or both of cardiovascular disease," wrote the Boston University School of Medicine
scientists. This deficiency "is associated with increased levels of total
cholesterol, low-density lipoprotein, increased production of proinflammatory factors, and increase thickness of the arterial wall."

Concerning type 2 diabetes and insulin resistance, this same
study's authors reviewed the science literature and concluded, "A
considerable body of evidence exists suggesting a link among reduced
testosterone plasma levels, type 2 diabetes, and insulin resistance."
Also noted were relationships between this hormone deficiency and
metabolic syndrome and erectile dysfunction.[10, 11]

Does having low T trigger all of the diseases and health conditions
listed below? The medical jury is still out debating its verdict on some
of these associations. For example, though some studies have found a
link between low T and metabolic syndrome, research continues on

whether low T triggers the syndrome or if it is having the syndrome that produces low T—another version of the old quandary: Which came first, the chicken or the egg?

While more scientific clarification is forthcoming, it's advisable for men to take notice and begin to treat these links as cautionary considerations when looking for their health concern causes, particularly because numerous authoritative studies have found that men with lower T levels die sooner than men with high T levels, and men with the highest T levels live healthier lives with fewer disabilities. Below are a few studies of these health concerns and their relation to low T.

Cardiovascular Disease—A 2011 study in the *Journal of Geriatric Cardiology* made this declaration: "Low levels of testosterone have been linked to a higher incidence of coronary artery disease. . . . We present some evidence from experimental and clinical studies that support the association between andropause and heart disease."[12]

Depression—Some psychiatric research into depressive illness have found a link to low testosterone. A study in the *Archives of General Psychiatry*, for instance, measured the testosterone levels in seventy-eight men, aged fifty-five and older, all without prior diagnosed depressive illness, and then these researchers did several years of follow-up testing with the group of men. Over that period, 21.7 percent of the low-testosterone men developed depression, compared to just 7 percent of the men with normal testosterone.[13]

Metabolic Syndrome—A cluster of conditions leading to diabetes and heart disease, characterized by having three or more of these measures: abdominal obesity, high triglyceride levels, high blood pressure, a fasting glucose of 100 mg/dL or greater, and an HDL cholesterol of less than 40 mg/dL in men. Numerous medical studies have identified low levels of total testosterone and low levels of sex hormone–binding globulin (SHBG) as being independent risk factors for developing metabolic syndrome.[14]

Mortality—In a 2008 published study of 794 men, ages fifty to ninety-one years, who had been medically surveyed over the previous eleven years and periodically had their testosterone levels measured, it was found that men with the lowest total testosterone levels were 40 percent more likely to die than the men who had the highest testosterone levels. This higher mortality rate was independent of metabolic syndrome, diabetes, and cardiovascular disease. In other words, low T is its own risk factor for dying at an earlier age than should be normal. This finding was confirmed six years later, in a European study that followed 2,599 men, aged forty to seventy-nine years, over four years, and found a fivefold higher risk of mortality for men with the lowest testosterone measured levels.[15, 16]

Nonalcoholic Fatty Liver Disease—It's a range of liver conditions afflicting people who drink little or no alcohol, characterized by a buildup of fat in liver cells preventing the liver from removing toxins from the blood. A survey of research in 2017 discovered that lower total testosterone levels are associated with men who have this chronic disorder, based on an analysis of sixteen clinical trials comprising 13,721 men. The higher the T levels in men, the lower their odds of getting NFLD.[17]

Stroke—Australian scientists evaluated testosterone levels in 3,690 men, aged seventy to eighty-nine years, and did follow-up with them over a six-year period. Those men with the highest levels of circulating testosterone or its metabolite, DHT, showed fewer strokes than men with lower levels of testosterone or its metabolite. The research team concluded in their published study that low T is a risk factor for having a stroke. No similar association was found for heart attacks.[18]

Type 2 Diabetes—In a review of results from forty-three studies, involving more than six thousand men, examining whether sex hormones play a role in type 2 diabetes, scientists writing in the *Journal of the American Medical Association* found that, on average, the studies showed "that men with higher testosterone levels had a 42 percent lower risk of type 2 diabetes." In other words, the lower your testosterone levels the greater your risk becomes of developing type 2 diabetes.[19]

Lifestyle Choices and Toxins Accelerate Aging

3

ONSET OF ANDROPAUSE and the depletion of a man's testosterone can be triggered, or even accelerated, by exposure to hormone-disrupting chemicals found in our food supply and consumer products and from the use of certain nonorganic personal care products. This chemical exposure may be resulting in unknown billions of dollars in additional health care costs. Scientists in the European Union attempted to calculate these costs for Europe in 2015, when they extrapolated toxicology evidence for male infertility, attributable to phthalate (a known hormone disrupter) exposure, along with other hormonal disruption impacts on male reproductive health. They found a 69 percent probability that lower testosterone in fifty-five- to sixty-four-year-old men, due to phthalate exposure, results in 24,800 associated deaths each year.[1]

It's already well documented that exposure to certain hormone-disruptive chemicals can trigger early menopause in women. A 2015 study, for example, found that the mean age of menopause onset was advanced by up to four years if a woman was exposed to any of three dozen chemicals classified as hormone disruptive. Similar research has yet to be conducted in men, but there is no rational reason why their exposure to such chemicals wouldn't also escalate the age at which they begin to experience hormone decline.[2]

A link has also been established between exposure to hormone disrupters and the obesity epidemic, an important contributor to rising health care costs, since obesity can produce type 2 diabetes and many other diseases that are expensive to treat. The hormone-disrupting chemicals inducing obesity are known as obesogens, molecules that distort the functioning of lipid metabolism in the body. (More on this phenomenon in a later chapter of this book.)[3]

When we start to closely look around us at the chemical soup our bodies are swimming in and absorbing, it can be daunting to consider. It becomes apparent that we must use our newfound awareness and knowledge to educate ourselves and others about these dangers, finding ways to protect ourselves and those we care about who depend on us to make responsible choices.

It's important to know, for example, how exposure to a range of pesticides can block male hormones and how drinking cow's milk can be problematic because it contains residues of hormone-disruptive chemicals, including growth hormones. Personal care products for men contain dozens of disrupters, which we will identify. Statins and other drugs magnify andropause symptoms, which can be a problem because almost a quarter of all men over forty years of age are on statin drugs to lower their cholesterol. Cholesterol helps to build testosterone, so if you lower your cholesterol too much, you limit the chemical building blocks available for testosterone production.

Hops used in beer contain estradiol, which interferes with testosterone production. Grapefruit consumption increases estrogen levels and undermines testosterone. Low vitamin D levels undermine testosterone, as well as other hormones, and don't overlook the role of nutrient deficiencies, such as having too little zinc in your diet.

All of these can be contributing factors to the onset of male hormone decline, reproductive disorders, and infertility. Four problem area sources, however, stand out from the hormone-disrupter crowd and deserve our closer scrutiny and vigilance.

Problem Source #1: Sugar Isn't a Male Hormone's Best Friend

If you want to efficiently and rapidly "steal" testosterone from a man's body, all you need to do is serve him foods and meals laden with sugar. It is a truism that the more sugar and carbs you eat, the more likely you'll develop insulin resistance or diabetes, which results in lower testosterone. By some estimates, up to 40 percent of men with type 2 diabetes have low testosterone.

One of the more starkly revealing studies showing the impact of sugar consumption on testosterone levels was done in 2013 and published in the science journal *Clinical Endocrinology*. A group of seventy-four men, ages nineteen to seventy-four, underwent a sampling of oral glucose accompanied by blood testing at intervals of 30, 60, 90, and 120 minutes. As part of the blood testing, measures were taken of fasting serum glucose, insulin, total testosterone, free testosterone, SHBG, leptin, and cortisol.

On average, glucose ingestion resulted in a 25 percent decrease in mean testosterone levels, and those levels remained suppressed at 120 minutes after absorption. This happened in both total and free testosterone levels. The impact of sugar on testosterone was so dramatic, that 15 percent of the men across the age ranges had their levels decrease until they were in the hypogonadal (andropausal) range at one or more of the time measurement points.

Further research amplified these findings and connected them to specific foods and drinks. For example, a 2018 study in the journal *Reproductive Biology Endocrinology* did blood testing with 545 men and also charted their consumption of sugar-sweetened beverages. Those men who drank the most of these sugar beverages had "significantly greater odds" of having low testosterone compared to the men who drank few (if any) of the beverages.

How and why this connection between sugar and testosterone exists was previously determined in a *Journal of Clinical Investigation* study in 2007, which found that consuming fructose and glucose can switch off a gene in men that regulates both testosterone and estrogen levels in the body, upsetting the delicate balance between those two hormones. Once that happens, obesity, erectile dysfunction, metabolic syndrome, and type 2 diabetes are often health impairments that follow in the wake, like pilot fish swimming after a shark.[4, 5, 6]

For more information about the impact of sugar on the health of all humans, not just men, we refer you to our book, *Sweet Disease: What Sugar and Artificial Sweeteners Are Doing to Your Health*.

Problem Source #2: Hormone Disrupters Hiding in Everyday Products

Some synthetic chemicals lurking in the environment and in common household products are mistaken by the human body as its own hormones. Once absorbed, these chemicals confuse and disrupt natural hormonal processes in the body, resulting in health problems and the triggering of many of the classic symptoms of andropause.

Six categories of hormone-disrupting chemicals have been identified by science studies as being present in cosmetics and personal care products. As detailed in the 2009 book, *Toxic Beauty*, by toxicologist and University of Illinois professor of environmental medicine Dr. Samuel S. Epstein, the six are preservatives, detergents, solvents, scents like tea tree oil and lavender, metalloestrogens, and ingredients in sunscreens.

Among preservatives, which are used in cosmetics and personal care products to prevent bacterial contamination and to stabilize ingredients, parabens and triclosan (as well as its chemically related cousin, triclocarban) are among the most studied and the most hormone disruptive.

Detergents, which are used as cleansers in products, include EDTA. Solvents, also known as plasticizers, dissolve other ingredients in water and include the commonly used phthalates, one of the more studied hormone disrupters. Lavender and tea tree oils are used in scented soaps and shampoos.

Metalloestrogens include metals such as aluminum and cadmium and appear in antiperspirants and sunscreens. Finally, sunscreens also often contain a range of disrupter chemicals such as benzophetone and oxybenzone, which have been detected in human breast milk, demonstrating how readily these disruptive chemicals are absorbed into the human body.[7]

To give you a few examples of what scientists have been finding, a research team at the University of California, Davis, did a study in 2007 that assessed the effects of antimicrobial products on human cells. Triclosan was found to inhibit testosterone "by more than 92 percent." Other parabens in those products were determined to inhibit testosterone by 40 percent, 33 percent, and 19 percent, prompting the scientists to conclude "the data presented in this report demonstrate that some widely used antimicrobial compounds have antiandrogenic properties" with "potential impact on human reproductive health."[8]

A review of the study literature on the hormone-disruptive effects of components of personal care products, conducted at the Virginia Commonwealth University, also produced evidence that high doses of phthalates can impair testosterone production by the testes, as can the antimicrobials triclocarban and triclosan. Though the review conceded that "select constituents (of personal care products) exhibit interactions with the endocrine system in the laboratory," the reviewers nonetheless were reluctant to directly link the products to hormone disruption.[9]

Oxybenzone, from sunscreens, was studied at the University of California, Riverside, in 2006, and they found that this hormone-disrupting chemical, which washes off sunbathers' bodies when they enter the ocean, had feminized male fish in two-thirds of two coastal fish species that were caught and then examined in the laboratory. A similar study in 2012, in Switzerland, found the same effects occurring in male zebrafish, after exposure to the same sunscreen chemical, raising the prospect that this phenomenon is also happening in male humans who apply the chemical to their skin.[10]

For up-to-date lists of safe and unsafe cosmetics and personal care products, a reputable resource is the Environmental Working Group: www.ewg.org.

Problem Source #3: Exposure to Pesticides Can Disrupt Your Hormones

If you fail to eat organic fruits and vegetables, you are exposing yourself to unhealthy levels of pesticide residues, many of which have been documented to be hormone disrupters.

Toxicologists at the University of London tested thirty-seven of the most widely used pesticides to assess their antihormonal activity, applying them to human cells and their hormone receptors, and found thirty of the pesticides mimicked or blocked male hormones. Until they were tested by these scientists, sixteen of the pesticides had never been found to be toxic to hormones before. Some of them were fungicides widely used on lettuce and strawberries. Of those toxins tested, the most potent hormone disrupter was fenirothion, an organophosphate insecticides widely applied to vegetables, rice, grains, and orchard fruits.

Another in this same family of pesticides, called Parathion, had previously been found to affect plasma testosterone in males. In animal lab tests, biologists writing in the science journal *Biocell* described how "plasma testosterone levels drop significantly at 8 days and recovered slowly at 40 days" after exposure to a single dose of Parathion. Exposure also negatively affected sperm count and sperm quality.

Men have two more reasons to be concerned about their exposure to hormone-disrupting pesticides on nonorganic fruits and vegetables. First, even many pesticides previously thought to be safe have been shown to disrupt hormones, based on cell in-vitro lab testing. Examples include flydioxonil and fenhexamid, which had been labeled "nonpersistent pesticides," meaning they weren't supposed to pose long-term harm to humans or the environment. "Even within permitted [legal] limits," these and other pesticides can "activate pathways affecting hormonal balance," concluded Austrian scientists in 2014, writing in the journal *Environmental Toxicology*.

Second, very little testing has been done to determine the impact of two or more of these toxic chemicals acting together synergistically, having impacts far more detrimental to hormones than any single chemical can exercise on its own. This point was driven home in 2017, when French scientists tested several previously untested pesticides (imazalil and propiconazole) and found them to "suppress testosterone to an extent greater than that seen with individual chemicals."

What all of these and related findings mean could have potentially profound implications for not just male hormonal health but all of human health management. Commercial food producers, the agricultural chemical industry, and government regulators remain resistant and far behind the scientific evidence in recognizing, and responding to, the health threats being identified as existing in our food supply.[11, 12, 13, 14]

Problem Source #4: Eat More Fast Food, Absorb More Toxins

Whether your fast food of choice is Burger King, McDonald's, or Taco Bell, or perhaps the highly processed prepackaged, microwavable offerings at convenience stores and gas stations, you are ingesting hormone-disrupting chemicals used in the plastic food-packaging wraps. The more fast food you eat, the more hormone disrupters you absorb, thus increasing your "body burden."

Statistics compiled and released in late 2018 by the National Center for Health Statistics (part of the Centers for Disease Control and Prevention) found that more than one in three Americans consume fast food on any given day. Men were more likely to eat fast food for lunch than women, and, contrary to what you might expect of poor people and their perceived reliance on cheap fast food, the percentage of adults who eat it actually increases as their family income increases.

These results were based on national surveys conducted among all age, racial, and ethnic groups. As you might suspect, younger people, aged twenty to thirty-nine years, had the highest fast-food consumption (44.9 percent of those surveyed), whereas adults aged sixty and over showed 24 percent eating fast food on a daily basis. The percentage consumption rates for the various racial groups were 42 percent for non-Hispanic blacks, 37 percent for non-Hispanic whites, 30 percent for Asians, and 35 percent for Hispanic adults.

Many scientific studies over the past few decades have documented how fast-food consumption increases a person's intake of unhealthy calories, fat, and sodium. Now we have research-based evidence that this consumption also dramatically escalates that person's body burden of hormone-disrupting chemicals.

A team of scientists at George Washington University in Washington, D.C., used health data collected on 8,877 Americans to evaluate their frequency of eating fast food, compared to their blood test results showing levels of phthalates, an industrial chemical used in fast-food wrappings. Phthalates are a confirmed hormone disrupter and leach out from plastic and paper packaging into the foods they wrap.

What the survey results showed was a dose-response relationship between fast-food intake and phthalate exposure. In other words, those who ate it had a 39 percent higher level of this chemical in their bodies than did persons who didn't regularly consume these convenience foods.

A subsequent study, done in 2018, at the University of California, Berkeley, did urinary spot sampling among 10,253 persons in the United States and measured their phthalate levels against their dining habits, which included all restaurants, not just fast-food joints. "We observed a consistent positive association between dining out and androgen-disrupter levels across the study population," the scientists concluded.

Those persons who were "high consumers of foods outside the home" had 55 percent higher phthalate hormone-disrupter levels in their bodies than persons who only consumed food at home. Cafeteria foods showed the highest association with phthalate body-burden levels, measuring 64 percent higher among adults who regularly ate in cafeterias, compared to adults who didn't.

It has long been known that certain foods are, by themselves, acting as hormone disrupters. A good example is licorice. A 2003 study discovered that eating licorice over the course of a week depletes a man's serum testosterone by 26 percent, thanks simply to the impact of the naturally occurring chemicals found in it. But what we now have in the United States and other highly industrialized countries is a situation in which some of the chemicals used in industrial processes, ostensibly to make life more comfortable and convenient for us, are instead undermining male hormonal development and fertility.

Beyond limiting your exposure to hormone disrupters by cutting fast foods from your diet, there are other steps you can take at home. Professor Leonardo Trasande, of the New York University Medical Center, who coauthored a study on the links between food container plastics and hypertension, recommends you do the following:

- Never cover your food with plastic wrap or put food in plastic containers and then microwave it, as that will leach the chemicals out into your meal.
- Never wash plastic food containers in a dishwasher; once again, plasticizer chemicals can leach out and contaminate other dishware.

Keep in mind that irrespective of whether you are male or female, these hormone-disruptive chemicals also can trigger illnesses and diseases in you that make the justification for using them— better living through chemistry—a sad joke on the future of our species.[15, 16, 17, 18, 19]

Other Disrupters: Smoking Pot Depletes Male Hormones

Marijuana is an androgen hormone antagonist! That certainly sounds scary, but what does it really mean? It's just that some of the chemicals found in the marijuana plant disrupt a man's androgen hormones, while having estrogen-like effects on the male body.

Evidence for this phenomenon first emerged in a 2005 science study in the journal *Toxicology*. Japanese scientists tested a series of marijuana extracts and found clear evidence that many "significantly inhibited" testosterone formation and "showed estrogen-like activity."

Add to that finding the prospect that for many pot users, getting the "munchies" from the high produces weight gain and that, in turn, can lead to obesity and metabolic syndrome, which further reduces testosterone levels.[20]

Another Potent Disrupter: Flame Retardants in Household Products

Duke University environmental health scientists recruited fifty men, between the ages of eighteen and fifty-four years old and tested their blood and also samples of their household dust, collected with vacuum cleaners.

High concentrations of two organophosphate flame retardant compounds, tris phosphate and triphenyl phosphate, were found in almost all of the dust samples from the fifty households (the two were detected in 96 percent and 98 percent of samples, respectively). These chemical compounds are known to be endocrine disrupters and yet are contained in furniture, electronics equipment, textiles, and plastics, from which they leach out into the surrounding environment. Based on the tests given, researchers were able to say the flame retardants were probably associated "with altered hormone levels and decreased semen quality in the men."[21]

An Antidote: Detox Hormone Disrupters Using Far-Infrared Saunas

Relying on saunas to sweat out toxins from the body dates back to Turkey, Nordic cultures, and the sweat lodges of Native American cultural practices, where the medicinal benefits of detoxification were understood intuitively, even if these benefits couldn't be explained scientifically.

Scientific research has caught up to traditional practices and found that both conventional saunas and newer techniques, like far-infrared saunas, which remove 78 percent or more toxins, convey numerous health benefits, including body detoxifying. The primary difference between the two is that far-infrared penetrates much more deeply into body tissues to release toxins that have accumulated in body fat.

At the Hippocrates Health Institute, we have made far-infrared saunas available to our guests for many years. We have personally seen and documented the many beneficial effects from detoxification, based on having conducted before-and-after blood testing to measure the "body burden" load of synthetic chemicals. So we know from observation and firsthand experience about its essential benefits.

Scientific studies have documented the effectiveness of sauna therapy in treating a range of health conditions: hypertension, cardiovascular disease, congestive heart failure, chronic obstructive pulmonary disease, chronic fatigue, chronic pain, joint mobility in patients with rheumatic disease, and even sleep disturbances. Some of these conditions, particularly fatigue and sleep disturbances, can be triggered by, or intensified by, the low testosterone and onset of andropause brought on by exposure to hormone-disrupting chemicals.

In a 2013 British study, for example, observing 138 patients who had mitochondrial dysfunction (mitochondria are the powerhouse for cells), a condition caused by the absorption of chemicals, one effect was chronic fatigue syndrome. Far-infrared saunas were a part of the treatment protocol and resulted in improvement by an average factor of four, which is rather impressive.[22, 23, 24, 25, 26, 27]

Lifting Brain "Fog"   4

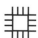

IF YOU NO LONGER CONSISTENTLY feel mental sharpness and you display increasingly frequent memory lapses, your fuzziness in thinking may be a result of low testosterone signaling the onset of andropause. It may even be a sign that your low T could trigger dementia.

Everyone has those periodic "senior moment" episodes when it seems like the brain neurons aren't firing effectively and we can't remember someone's name, or we don't feel as if we are performing mental tasks up to normal levels. This brain "fog" is part of being human and being occasionally fallible, rather than just a normal part of aging. But deterioration in male hormones, particularly testosterone, exceeds "normal" and expected boundaries, and becomes a cause for concern, when a man's ability to mentally function can no longer be taken for granted.

Scientific study evidence paints both broad brush strokes and finely detailed pictures of the impact hormonal declines exact on brain function in men, affecting decision-making, short- and long-term memory, mental clarity, and, of course, the risks for developing dementia and Alzheimer's disease.

Evidence for Dementia and Alzheimer's

"Lower than normal testosterone levels have also been detected in patients prior to the onset of [Alzheimer's disease], as well as in younger late-onset male AD patients," concluded a 2007 study in the *Journal of Alzheimer's Disease.*[1]

An even larger and more recent study done in Australia, involving 4,069 men who were assessed over a ten-year period, concluded that "lower plasma total and calculated free testosterone were associated with increased risk of developing dementia."[2]

Evidence for Memory Impairment

To study the link between serum testosterone levels and measureable declines in memory performance, scientists at the National Institute on Aging recruited 407 men, aged fifty to ninety-one years, and assessed them over a ten-year period using cognitive testing and blood testing. The results were clear: men with the lowest testosterone "had significantly lower scores on measures of memory and visuospatial performance and a faster rate of decline in visual memory."[3]

Evidence for Impaired Decision-Making

Canadian scientists evaluated testosterone levels and cognitive executive (decision-making) in fifty-four healthy older men and found "significant associations between working memory function and both free and bioavailable testosterone levels, suggesting that an optimal hormone level may exist for maximal performance on tasks of executive/frontal lobe functioning."[4]

Two Underreported Reasons for Mild to Severe Cognitive Decline

Have your vitamin D levels checked.

A team of nutritional and neurological scientists tested 382 people, over a five-year period, to measure both their cognitive abilities and their vitamin D levels, which are essential to bone health. These test subjects ranged in age from their sixties to their nineties and included whites, African Americans, and Hispanics. What the testing showed was that a correlation existed between vitamin D in the body and cognitive decline over the five-year testing period. "On average, people with low vitamin D declined two to three times as fast as those with adequate vitamin D," observed Professor Joshua Miller, a study coauthor from the Rutgers School of Environmental and Biological Sciences.

Though 54 percent of the Caucasians and 70 percent of the Hispanics and African Americans had low blood levels of vitamin D, low levels signaled a greater cognitive loss irrespective of a person's ethnicity or race. This cognitive decline was measured based on testing for episodic memory and executive functioning of the brain. The reason for this vitamin/cognition link is not entirely clear.

Anyone experiencing chronic symptoms of cognitive decline should have their blood tested for vitamin D. If levels are low, the study authors recommend vitamin D supplements, particularly if you are more than sixty years of age.[5]

Second, check the prescription and over-the-counter medications you take.

A class of drugs known as anticholinergics, which help to contract and relax muscles and are used as sleep aids, nighttime cold medications, and treatments for depression and Parkinson's disease, have been found to raise the risk for brain impairment and cognitive decline.

More than four hundred persons were studied, some anticholinergic drug users and some not, in research at the Indiana University School of Medicine, and every eighteen months they had MRIs done for brain structure changes and PET scans done to measure brain metabolism. The results, released in 2016, were dramatic.

It was clear that the anticholinergic drug users had lower levels of glucose metabolism, a measure for brain activity, and reduced brain volume, as well as worse performances than the non-drug group on tests for short-term memory, verbal reasoning, and problem solving, the so-called executive functions of the brain. Generally, cognitive problems started showing up in the anticholinergic group within sixty days of continuous use.

A more recent study, published in the *British Medical Journal* in 2018, examined 40,777 persons, aged sixty-five to ninety-nine, who had been diagnosed with dementia, and compared them to 283,933 persons (the control group) who didn't have diagnosed dementia. Daily doses of anticholinergic drugs were compiled and compared to both study groups.

"A robust association between some classes of anticholinergic drugs and future dementia incidence was observed," noted the study authors. These greater-risk drugs were used as antidepressants, for urological purposes, and as anti-Parkinson treatments.[6, 7]

Solution Options to Prevent, Slow, or Reverse Cognitive Decline

A Combination of Aerobic Exercise and Diet

Duke University scientists took 160 male and female adults, aged fifty-five years and older, and divided them up into four lifestyle intervention groups of forty persons each. They assessed their executive (decision-making) brain functions over a six-month period.

One group did aerobic exercise, which involved brisk walking, or cycling for thirty-five minutes a day, three times a week.

A second group adhered to a DASH (Dietary Approaches to Stop Hypertension) diet, which includes eating more fruits and vegetables, limiting sugar and sodium intake, cutting back on all foods high in saturated fats.

The third group did a combination of aerobic exercise and DASH diet.

A fourth group only engaged in health education.

Results published in a 2018 edition of the science journal *Neurology* found the exercise regimen to have a sizably favorable impact, but "the largest improvements [in executive brain function] were observed for participants randomized to the combined AE [aerobic exercise] and DASH diet group."

"The results showed that controlled aerobic activity within a very short period of time can have a significant impact on the part of the brain that keeps people taking care of themselves, paying their bills and the like," commented Dr. Richard Isaacson, director of the Alzheimer's Prevention Clinic at Weill Cornell Medicine.

Even more remarkably, the combination diet and exercise group was estimated to have *reversed* their brain aging by at least nine years! By contrast, the control group, who received only health education, experienced an executive function decline of six months in their test scores, which was the expected age-related decline without a lifestyle intervention.[8]

Improving Fitness Helps Reverse Brain Shrinkage

To determine whether initiating a fitness routine could reverse both neurodegeneration and the shrinkage of gray matter that occurs with age, University of Maryland School of Public Health scientists brought together a group of sixty-one to eighty-eight-year-old people who had been previously physically inactive. They were a mix of mentally healthy as well as patients with mild cognitive impairment.

Study participants did moderate intensity walking on a treadmill, four times a week, over a twelve-week study period. Before-, during-, and after-study measurements were taken of their brain cortex thickness, an outer layer brain area that typically atrophies during cognitive impairment and early Alzheimer's stages.

Among both the healthy and the mildly impaired participants, those who showed the most fitness improvements over twelve weeks also measured the greatest growth in their brain's cortical layer. Neural efficiency also improved, including memory recall.

"Many people think it is too late to intervene with exercise once a person shows symptoms of memory loss," commented study coauthor, Dr. J. Carson Smith, in a 2015 interview. "But our data suggest that exercise may have a benefit in this early stage of cognitive decline."[9]

The Mediterranean Diet Slows Brain Aging and Decline

A Mediterranean diet, characterized by increased consumption of fruits and vegetables and a decrease or elimination of dairy, meat, and sugars, bestows numerous benefits to the human brain and cognition, according to numerous science studies, making it a "brain food" diet.

In a 2015 study in the journal *Neurology*, 674 elderly adults without dementia had their diet examined through food questionnaires, then underwent MRI brain scans to measure total gray matter volume, mean cortical thickness, and other markers for brain health. Results showed that "among older adults, Mediterranean

Diet adherence was associated with less brain atrophy, with an effect similar to 5 years of aging."[10]

Similarly, a 2016 article in the science journal *Frontiers of Nutrition* reviewed fifteen years of studies on the Mediterranean diet and found eighteen that demonstrated how adherence to the diet "is associated with slower rates of cognitive decline, reduced conversion to Alzheimer's disease, and improvements in cognitive functioning. The specific cognitive domains that were found to benefit were memory (delayed recognition, long-term, and working memory), executive function, and visual constructs."[11]

A Diet to Slow Brain Aging by 7.5 Years

A 2015 study funded by the National Institute on Aging compared the Mediterranean diet and the DASH diet, both discussed above, to a hybrid dietary regimen called MIND, developed specifically to help brain functioning over time among those at risk for dementia and Alzheimer's. Researchers at Rush University Medical Center enrolled in the study 960 persons, an average of eighty-one years of age, who were free of dementia. For nearly five years, they were assessed by the medical team with cognitive ability tests in five areas—episodic memory, working memory, semantic memory, visuospatial ability, and perceptual speed. They also filled out food questionnaires to assess their adherence to the MIND diet over the study period.

The MIND diet includes ten brain-healthy food groups, such as daily green leafy vegetables, nuts, berries, beans, whole grains, and olive oil. The diet eliminates red meats, butter and stick margarine, cheese, pastries, sweets, and fried or fast foods of any sort.

It had already been shown in previous studies that adherence to the Mediterranean and DASH diets reduced risks for Alzheimer's disease, as well as for cardiovascular disease. This MIND diet tweaked these other two diets in various ways. For instance, blueberries were included and emphasized because studies have shown them to be a potent brain protective food when eaten on their own.

At the end of the nearly five-year study period, researchers found the MIND diet "substantially slowed cognitive decline" over all five of their cognitive measures of brain function. In fact, they were able to estimate that participants with the greatest adherence to the diet took 7.5 years of cognitive decline with aging off, compared to those with no, or the least adherence, to the diet.

Three years later, a study review was released examining subsequent research comparing the MIND diet with the DASH and Mediterranean diets. It concluded, "Results suggest that higher adherence to a healthy dietary pattern is associated with preservation of brain structure and function as well as slower cognitive decline, with the MIND diet substantially slowing cognitive decline, over and above the Mediterranean and DASH diets."[12, 13]

Maintaining a Mindfulness Meditation Practice

In a series of 2015 studies on the health benefits of having a regular mindfulness meditation practice, researchers recruited persons aged fifty-five to seventy-five years old and had them engage in a regular mindfulness practice over eight weeks, as their brain activity was periodically measured while doing cognitive tasks. As the research team reported, "the results show that engaging in just over ten minutes of mindfulness practice five times per week resulted in significant improvements" in general brain task performance. The results indicate that the practice "may be a useful strategy for counteracting cognitive decline associated with aging."

Observed study coauthor Peter Malinowski, "The results show that the meditation practice improved the ability to maintain attention on a rather repetitive task—on indicating correctly how many words appeared on [a] screen. It also shows that at a mean age of sixty-five years it is not too late—picking up meditation at that point can lead to rapid cognitive improvements. If we consider that the meditation practice consisted of focusing on the sensation of one's own breath, the results seem even more remarkable."[14]

Brain Enhancements by Elevating Magnesium

Scientists at MIT, in 2010, developed a treatment for older adults with cognitive impairment using magnesium L-threonate supplementation, which subsequent studies found can reverse the symptoms of brain-aging mental fog.

One of the clinical trials involved older adults, fifty to seventy years of age, who were given either the magnesium supplement or a placebo for twelve weeks and had their cognitive ability periodically evaluated. "Overall cognitive ability improved significantly relative to placebo," the research team concluded. Study subjects had impaired executive functions in their brain, and those given the supplement "nearly restored their impaired executive function" in just twelve weeks.

This magnesium supplement seems to work by increasing the density of synapses in the brain, which act as communication connections between brain cells. The supplement also seemed to help treat those study subjects who had sleep disorders.[15]

Testosterone Supplementation for Cognitive Decline

Other scientific evidence for natural solutions to cognitive decline include the favorable results of clinical trials showing the positive effects of testosterone supplementation on men with impaired cognitive functioning. Not all studies have found testosterone replacement therapy to be effective in improving brain function and lifting brain fog. However, as a 2016 study review from the University of Colorado School of Medicine framed it, these testosterone/cognition studies, taken together, "have had a wide range of results. The variability in outcomes is likely related, in part, to the lack of consensus on methods for testosterone measurement and supplementation and, in part, to the disparate measures of cognitive function used in randomized controlled studies. Despite the limitations imposed by such inconsistent methods, promising associations have been found between cognition and testosterone supplementation."[16]

Among those studies finding a positive correlation between improved cognitive ability and testosterone supplementation, the following stand out as offering encouragement and hope to men in andropause:

In the science journal *Neurology*, University of Washington Medical School researchers evaluated twenty-five healthy men, aged fifty to eighty years, over six weeks as they were injected with 100 mg testosterone (or were given a placebo) and conducted cognitive assessments. Compared to the placebo group, those given testosterone supplementation show "significant improvements in cognition for spatial memory, spatial ability, and verbal memory."[17]

A larger and longer study was conducted by Australian scientists in 2016, using forty-four test subjects evaluated over twenty-four weeks. Men in the supplementation group received 50 mg a day of a testosterone cream called AndroForte, applied to the scrotum. Neuropsychological measures were taken four times during the six-month study period. Compared to the control group, those given supplementation showed "a modest improvement in global cognition."[18]

Handling Depression and Mood Changes

5

I F A MAN REGULARLY BECOMES IRRITABLE for no apparent reason, or releases anger at the slightest provocation, or develops depressive moods previously uncharacteristic for him, he may be suffering from the hormonal imbalances caused by age-triggered andropause. As discussed earlier in this book, we call this phenomenon Irritable Male Syndrome.

It was first identified in the scientific literature in 2001, described as "a behavioral state of nervousness, irritability, lethargy and depression that occurs in adult male mammals following withdrawal of testosterone." In the animal kingdom, Irritable Male Syndrome is characterized as a negative mood state in seasonally breeding mammals, at the end of the mating season, in which "the animals appear agitated and fearful, and the incidence of physical wounding owing to fractious inter-male fighting peaks at this time."[1]

In male humans, a loss of testosterone seems to activate the "fight or flight response" as well, though studies are sparse on the extent to which this hormonal deprivation initiates violence, either male on male or male on female. We can imagine, however, the possible usefulness of initiating science studies examining whether the male instigators of mass shootings, random criminal acts, and "crimes of passion" violence are, in fact, being triggered by hormonal imbalances, becoming the most extreme examples of Irritable Male Syndrome.

Some studies have found evidence of an association between testosterone imbalances and suicidal behavior in men. Ironically, evidence seems to suggest that "suicidal behavior in adolescents and young adults is associated with high testosterone levels, whereas suicidality in older men is associated with decreased testosterone secretion," concluded a 2013 study.[2]

Follow-up research done in 2016, reported that "both high and low testosterone levels may play a role in suicidal behavior in man of any age," not just among young and old men. Though more experiments need to be conducted, this possible connection opens up an entire new realm of research into the source and triggers for not just suicides among men but all forms of hostility and aggression producing violence in the human species.[3]

General depression is another mental health condition in men potentially connected to a hormone imbalance. As we pointed out elsewhere in this book, when a man comes to a physician showing symptoms of depression, the physician will usually prescribe an antidepressant drug, rather than check for low testosterone, which is also a trigger for depression. Drugs are what most mainstream physicians are trained to reach for first.

In a 2015 study of 521 men, half of them showed clinical symptoms of andropause (with low testosterone), and among those men, symptoms of depression were much higher than among the non-andropausal men, prompting the study authors to conclude, "There is a direct association between andropause symptoms and depression."[4]

Still another 2015 study, this one involving 196 middle-aged and elderly men (aged forty to eighty years), found "more severe depression symptoms associated with low testosterone." The highest correlation of all was seen in prediabetic men with low testosterone, compared to healthy men.[5]

Readers of this book can help educate their own physicians about the importance of proper diagnostic testing of testosterone levels as a first step in treating depression and related mood disorders. Below are a series of natural solution options for treating the symptoms of depression, which, taken together, may provide you with a realistic practical combination of remedies to try, given your own preferences and needs, to forestall the use of pharmaceutical antidepressants as a first line of defense.

Natural Solution Option: Mindfulness Meditation

Researchers at the U.S. Department of Defense's Deployment Health Clinical Center surveyed the results of fifty-two study reviews and randomized clinical trials in 2016, investigating whether mindfulness meditation training and practice is effective in treating depressive disorders and posttraumatic stress. "Mindfulness-based interventions are safe, portable, cost-effective, and can be recommended as an adjunct to standard care or self-management strategy for major depressive disorder and PTSD," the health researchers concluded.[6]

Natural Solution Option: Vigorous Physical Exercise

Norwegian psychologists surveyed twenty-three randomized controlled trials of using physical exercise as a depression treatment—nearly one thousand study participants were involved—and compared the findings of all these studies. "Exercise compared to no intervention yielded a large and significant effect size," the scientists concluded. "Exercise had a moderate and significant effect compared to usual care [for depression]." When combined with an antidepressant medication, exercise also yielded a significant effect.[7]

Researchers at the Medical University of South Carolina, writing in the *International Journal of Psychiatry*, went even further in extolling the virtues of vigorous exercise to treat depression. They observed that "exercise compares favorably to antidepressant medications as a first-line treatment for mild to moderate depression."[8]

How frequent and intense should the exercise be to relieve symptoms of depression? Study research indicates that vigorous aerobic exercise, at least three to five times per week, at least thirty minutes per session, should help do the trick.[9]

Natural Solution Option: St. John's Wort Supplementation

A flowering shrub called St. John's wort has long been used as a natural herbal supplement for treating the symptoms of depression. Many dozens of science studies have been conducted on whether the herb is as effective as advertised. Generally, the results have been positive, though it doesn't seem to work for everyone (but what does?).

According to the National Institutes of Health, "A 2008 review of 29 international studies suggested that St. John's wort may be better than a placebo and as effective as different standard prescription antidepressants for major depression of mild to moderate severity. St. John's wort also appeared to have fewer side effects than standard antidepressants."[10]

Natural Solution Option: Eating a Healthy Diet

Let thy food be thy medicine, said the ancient Greek medical philosopher Hippocrates, and that seems true for all health conditions, including moodiness and depression. Diet quality, particularly a plant-based diet, is the key to helping prevent and treat the symptoms of depression. In 2018, the *Journal of Affective Disorders* published a study review that compared the results on the diet and depression link from twenty-four separate studies. "Adherence to a high-quality diet [such as the Mediterranean diet] was associated with a lower risk of depressive symptoms over time," the study review concluded from the evidence.[11]

The lower your intake of animal foods, the lower becomes your risk of depression, another survey of the scientific literature advised in 2017. Specifically, this study review cited red and processed meats, refined grains, sweets, most dairy products such as butter, and high-fat gravy as foods you need to avoid to lower the risk of depression or a recurrence of depression.[12]

Why do these specific foods trigger depression? The reason seems to do with the level of inflammation in the body caused by their consumption. The more often you eat these foods, the more chronic inflammation you inflict on your body tissues and organs.[13]

Natural Solution Option: DHEA Supplementation

A steroid hormone, DHEA (dehydroepiandrosterone), is produced by the adrenal gland and plays a role in protecting brain functions, including mood stabilization. Its secretions decline with age.

Science research has shown that declining DHEA levels not only play a role in depression but also result in the brain shrinkage that accompanies major depression. A 2013 study conducted at the University of Michigan's Department of Psychiatry, investigated which specific areas of the brain are influenced by DHEA in mitigating depression.

Patients in the study were given 400 mg of DHEA each day while undergoing fMRI scans of their brains. It was discovered that DHEA reduced activity in the amygdala and hippocampus brain areas, reducing negative emotional effects. "Our results provide initial neuroimaging evidence that DHEA may be useful as a pharmacological intervention for these conditions [negative emotions and depression]," the research team concluded.[14]

Natural Solution Option: Testosterone Replacement Therapy

In a review of the science study literature, Florida State University scientists concluded in 2014, that "testosterone may have protective benefits against anxiety and depression." While they were unable to provide the "precise underlying mechanisms" for how replacing lost testosterone can have protective benefits, they speculated that it may be the result of a complex interplay between brain regions, neural circuits, and cellular and molecular pathways.[15]

A body of previous research had found, according to the *International Journal of Impotence Research*, striking evidence that "testosterone replacement was associated with improved mood and well-being, and reduced fatigue and irritability. Notably, in one of these clinical trials, the investigators continued to follow 123 men on testosterone replacement for three years and reported that the improvements in mood persisted."[16]

Combating Bone and Joint Degeneration

6

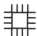

WHEN BONE FRACTURES OCCUR more easily and frequently with age, and you are experiencing chronic bone and joint weakness, including low back pain, it may be due to low testosterone levels. Untreated, this condition can lead to osteoporosis (the loss of bone density and mass) or to rheumatoid arthritis (an inflammatory disease of the joints).

Testosterone seems to play an anti-inflammatory role in the body, particularly the male body, helping to protect bone and joint health. DHEA (dehydroespiandrosterone sulfate—another hormone that declines with age) levels appear to play a supporting role in preventing painful joint and bone conditions.[1] While study evidence suggests that both men and women who have rheumatoid arthritis show lower levels of testosterone in their blood compared to healthy people, it's a linkage factor that seems to be more pronounced in males, if only because they had much higher levels of the hormone than women to begin with. Swedish scientists documented this phenomenon in 2014, in a study for the *Annals of Rheumatoid Disease*. They measured blood testosterone in 104 men over a twelve-year period and saw, as hormone levels went into a steady decline, that this predicted whether the study participants would have a greater risk for developing the disease.[2]

It used to be, until relatively recently, that osteoporosis was treated as primarily a disease women experience later in life. We're not sure why men were ignored in this health equation, but sometime in the early twenty-first century, it was as if a collective light bulb flickered on within the medical profession, which finally began to recognize, in the words of one science research team, "that osteoporosis constitutes an inseparable element of getting old for men as well."[3]

For women, estrogen deficiency in menopause can trigger the loss of bone density, resulting in osteoporosis, a phenomenon well known among scientists for decades. It's now more firmly understood that testosterone decline also affects bone quality, raising fracture risk.[4]

One reason why scientists finally started to recognize the testosterone and bone density link in men was the impact they were seeing of androgen deprivation therapy in treating prostate cancer. "Osteoporosis is a common consequence of androgen deprivation therapy for prostate cancer," observed a 2011 study in the journal *Maturitas*. "Up to 20% of men on androgen deprivation therapy for localized prostate cancer will fracture within 5 years."[5]

A man's amount of free circulating testosterone, as opposed to total testosterone levels, seems to be most predictive of whether the man will develop low bone mineral density leading to fractures and osteopenia (bone weakness that can lead to osteoporosis). This was the finding of a 2009 study, published in the science journal *Clinical Endocrinology*, which examined 1,185 men, aged twenty to ninety years, and discovered that men with the lowest free testosterone had a four times higher risk than men with the highest levels.[6]

So now that we know more clearly the connection between male hormones and bone and joint health, what natural treatment alternatives exist for men?

We know of compelling scientific evidence for the effectiveness of a range of botanicals (plant extracts) and key nutrients that reduce inflammation in the joints, increase bone density, and even repair some of the damage. These range from the botanicals white mulberry, cutch tree, and Chinese skullcap to the nutrients vitamin D, calcium, zinc, magnesium, and boron. It's possible for you to create a modifying therapy for bone disease from combinations of these healing agents.

Natural Solution Option: White Mulberry and Cutch Tree

Called *Morus alba*, the bark of the white mulberry tree has long been used by ancient cultures as an anti-inflammatory. Late twentieth-century science determined that this tree bark and its roots contain high levels of flavonoids, and more in-depth research drew connections from consumption of this inflammatory with the protection of joints and the relief of joint pain.

The other anti-inflammatory, known scientifically as *Acacia catechu*, otherwise known as cutch tree, is a South Asian tree, but it's considered a part of the legume family. Like beans, the heartwood and bark of this tree contain catechins, the flavonoid valued for its healing bioactive powers, particularly as an anti-inflammatory.

These two botanical compounds were thoroughly studied in 2016 and 2017 for their use in relieving pain and inflammation of the joints caused by osteoarthritis. The first extensive study occurred in lab animals and found the two compounds had effects similar to high-dose ibuprofen, making it appropriate for use in treating arthritis.[7]

A second lab animal study combined extracts of white mulberry and the cutch tree as a targeted therapy for osteoarthritis. A synergistic effect was observed (the two compounds interacted in ways more powerful than any single compound did on its own), and the result was "significant improvements" in cartilage and bone health and an up to 41 percent reduction in pain sensitivity.[8]

Finally, a study done with 135 human subjects, over twelve weeks, tested a blend of the two compounds for treatment of osteoarthritis of the knee. Not only did range of motion and walking distance improve, along with reductions in pain and discomfort, but the science team was able to conclude that "early intervention [with the compound combination] aimed at reducing bone and cartilage degradation . . . may help to prevent joint cartilage damage."[9]

Natural Solution Option: Vitamin D Supplementation

Vitamin D3, one of the two main forms of vitamin D, "has been shown to be important in bone health and can influence rheumatoid arthritis disease activity," observed a 2018 study in the *International Journal of Rheumatoid Disease.*[10]

Because Vitamin D is also involved in regulating the balance of calcium and phosphorous in the human body, both important to bone health, this vitamin's role as an anti-inflammatory reaches critical importance in males when andropause begins affecting bones and cartilage. A study done in 2013, published in the journal *Osteoporosis International*, assessed eighty men, average age of sixty-nine years, with low bone mineral density and gave them vitamin D supplements as part of their treatment protocol. The result was, the Canadian scientists concluded, "use of vitamin D was associated with improved bone mineral density in the lumbar spine in year 1" of the study.[11]

Natural Solution Option: Testosterone Replacement Therapy

Florida scientists associated with the Veterans Affairs Medical Center gave sixty men, with an average age of sixty years, fifty-two weeks of treatment with testosterone enanthate, an injectable compound, to test the beneficial effects on their musculoskeletal structure. The study finding was that the compound "significantly increases muscle strength and bone mineral density and reduces body fat without causing prostate enlargement."[12]

Japanese scientists tested the effects of testosterone replacement therapy on seventy-four men with a clinical diagnosis of osteoporosis or osteopenia (a less severe form of bone loss and weakness). They were given 250 mg of testosterone enanthate injections every four weeks for twelve months. At study's end, the men showed "significant increase in bone mineral density."[13]

Finally, a 2017 study, published in the *Journal of the American Medical Association Internal Medicine*, involved the use of testosterone gel applied to 211 men, average age of seventy-two years, for twelve months. Bone mineral density in the spine and hips of these men was measured before and after testosterone administration. The findings were conclusive: "Testosterone treatment for 1 year of older men with low testosterone significantly increased bone mineral density and estimated bone strength."[14]

Rebuilding Muscle Mass   7

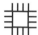

A N AVERAGE MAN'S LEAN BODY MASS decreases by about 10 percent every decade due to aging and a lower production of testosterone. As a man loses muscle mass, he gains even more body fat, resulting in less circulating testosterone, which further compounds the problem.

Science studies have directly linked testosterone loss with age to muscle wasting, loss of strength and power, and diminished overall exercise capacity. All of this loss of physical function contributes to an overall frail condition that invites a further decline in health.

Frailty, along with all of its potential disability for broken hips from falls, is one direct result of losing skeletal muscle mass. In a study of 461 men, sixty years and older, Swiss scientists found that low free testosterone was a key factor "associated with a significantly increased odds of frailty," based on five criteria for assessing someone as frail. Men with free testosterone levels below 243 pmol/L, had the highest increased odds of becoming frail.[1]

A consequence of low testosterone in older men can be anemia (iron-poor or "tired" blood), resulting in weakness that can be another contributing factor to a diminishment of muscle strength and function, triggering muscle wasting. In a 2017 study involving twenty-three scientists from a dozen universities, a group of 788 men, sixty-five years and older, were evaluated for their testosterone levels and symptoms of anemia. "Among men with low testosterone

levels," the science team concluded, "testosterone treatment significantly increased the hemoglobin levels of those with unexplained
anemia as well as those with anemia from known causes."[2]

Natural Solution: Resistance Strength Training

Doing weight training, and doing it consistently, can increase testosterone production, which builds lean muscle and depletes fat.
Scientific evidence even shows which resistance exercises are most
effective, how often they need to be done for best results, and what
dietary changes need to be made to supplement these results.

Doing resistance training with weights, particularly if you focus
on working out your legs, not only directly builds muscle but also
triggers the release of testosterone (and growth hormone), which
helps to build even more muscle to counteract the effects of aging.

As the science journal *Sports Medicine* declared, "Resistance exercise
has been shown to elicit a significant hormonal response. . . . Anabolic
hormones such as testosterone and the superfamily of growth hormones (GH) have been shown to be elevated during 15–30 minutes
of post-resistance exercise."[3]

Irrespective of whether a man is sixty-two years old or thirty years
old, heavy resistance training elevates total testosterone. That result
was clearly shown in a *Journal of Applied Physiology* study in which
two groups of men, one group thirty years of age on average and the
other sixty-two years on average, had their blood measured over ten
weeks of a resistance training program. Though the younger group
demonstrated higher total and free testosterone levels than the older
men, this latter group also experienced "a significant increase in total
testosterone."[4]

Something else to factor in when using resistance training to elevate testosterone is the impact of rest intervals between exercise sets.
This was demonstrated in a study of men doing high-intensity bench
presses. Resting for one minute versus three minutes in between each
bench press set had different impacts on testosterone levels, as measured with blood testing. The longer rest period "promoted a long-

lasting elevation for both total testosterone and free testosterone," compared to the one-minute duration rest period.[5]

Studies have even been done comparing the effects on testosterone of resistance training between lean men and obese men. California State University researchers took ten physically active obese males (with 36 percent and more body fat) and ten lean men (less than 12 percent body fat) and put them through a resistance training protocol of six sets of ten repetitions per leg, while taking blood samples before, during, and after. Increases in testosterone were similar in both body types.[6]

Natural Solution: Apples and Green Tomatoes

During a research study by a team from the Iowa Veterans Affairs Medical Center, investigating the molecular mechanisms of age-related skeletal muscle weakness and atrophy, several molecules were identified that can "significantly reduce age-related deficits in skeletal muscle strength, quality and mass."

These two molecules with potential therapeutic intervention applications are ursolic acid (found in apples) and tomatidine (derived from green tomatoes). Once inside the human body, these molecules activate something known as an activating transcription factor 4 (ATF4), to act on skeletal muscle and reduce the impact of aging. By reducing ATF4 activity in the body, these two molecules enable skeletal muscle to recover from the effects of aging.

"Many of us know from our own experiences that muscle weakness and atrophy are big problems as we become older," commented Dr. Christopher Adams, a senior author of the study. "These problems have a major impact on our quality of life and health. Based on these results, ursolic acid and tomatidine appear to have a lot of potential as tools for dealing with muscle weakness and atrophy during aging."

Work is now under way by Adams and colleagues "to translate ursolic acid and tomatidine into foods, supplements, and pharmaceuticals that can help preserve or recover strength and muscle mass as people grow older," according to a University of Iowa release statement.[7, 8]

Natural Solution: Nicotinamide Riboside Supplementation

Though studies so far have only been done in lab animals, a molecule called NAD, found in every cell in the human body and used to power metabolism, holds potential for rebuilding and maintaining muscle mass. NAD declines with age and scientists know it's important for muscle development and regeneration. In a 2016 study, done by a team of scientists from the University of Pennsylvania, a precursor of NAD called nicotinamide riboside was administered to lab animals that had lost skeletal muscle. This muscle deficit was rapidly restored in animals given the supplement, prompting the research team to write; it could "play a critical role" in "maintaining muscle mass and function."[9]

Natural Solution: Testosterone Replacement Therapy

Replacement of lost testosterone in the male body "increases lean body mass and decreases fat mass," declared a study by researchers from the UCLA School of Medicine, "and the magnitude of the changes induced by testosterone are correlated with dose. Older men are as responsive to the anabolic effects of testosterone on the muscle as young men."[10]

Scientific studies examining this linkage in detail have been numerous over the past two decades. For example, in 2012 scientists applied a testosterone treatment gel to thirty-eight men, aged sixty to seventy-eight years, all of whom had low to normal bioavailable testosterone levels, and measured the effects on their insulin sensitivity, metabolism, body composition, and lipids. Their finding: "testosterone therapy increased muscle mass."[11]

In a three-year study, whose results were published in 2017, healthy men aged sixty years and older, with total testosterone levels of 100 to 400 Ng/dL, were divided into two groups: one that received a testosterone gel daily, and the other that received a placebo gel. At the end of three years, men in the testosterone treatment group showed "significantly greater improvements in stair-climbing power, muscle mass, and power," according to the research team from seven U.S. universities.[12]

A 2018 study, published in *The Lancet*, divided 790 men, aged sixty-five years and older, into two study groups: one that received testosterone gel every day for twelve months, and a placebo group that received no special treatment. Both groups were tested before, during, and after the study time frame for their physical mobility and their walking speed. The research findings were clear: "Testosterone-treated men reporting mobility limitation showed significantly more improvement in walking distance and walking ability."[13]

Finally, another 2018 study compared whether injecting testosterone into the body was more effective than applying a testosterone gel in building muscle. By comparing the findings from thirty-one randomized clinical trials, University of Florida scientists determined that intramuscular injections of testosterone "were 3–5 times greater" in their positive effects on muscle mass and muscle strength than the use of transdermal gel formulations.[14]

Slowing Hair Thinning   8

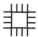

BEGINNING AROUND FORTY YEARS OF AGE, many men experience hair loss that has a visible impact on the head, chest, legs, under the arms, and even in the thickness of pubic hair. Simultaneously, these men may be growing unwanted hair in the ears and nose, sticking up and out until they resemble porcupines.

By the age of fifty, estimates are that half of all males will be losing some (if not most) of their hair. Most instances of male-pattern hair loss, as the condition is known, apparently begin with a variation in a gene, AR, which provides instructions "for making a protein called an androgen receptor," according to the U.S. National Library of Medicine. "Androgen receptors allow the body to respond appropriately to dihydrotestosterone (DHT) and other androgens."[1] Other causes for hair loss may include anemia, a thyroid problem, blood thinner medications, effects of radiation and chemotherapy treatments, chronic stress, insufficient nutrients in your diet, or even keeping your hair tied back in a ponytail or braids for years.

Back to DHT: it's made from testosterone in the body using an enzyme, and it's important to the body in maintaining the health of hair follicles. When too much of it is produced, it can cause acne and stimulate the growth of prostate cells, resulting in that nagging and uncomfortable condition called BPH—benign prostatic hyperplasia.

With your hair follicles, your genetics determine sensitivity to that AR gene, and that sensitivity influences whether your body's producing too much DHT will cause hair loss.

A question thus arises: Since DHT "drives both hair loss and the growth of prostate cells, do men with hair loss (androgenic alopecia) have an increased risk of prostate cancer?" asked Harvard Medical School researchers. "Perhaps, according to scientists in Australia. They evaluated 1,446 men who were diagnosed with moderate to high-grade prostate cancer before age seventy and compared them with 1,390 men of the same age who were free of the disease. The researchers looked at each man's scalp, then used sophisticated statistical methods to see if there was a link between hair loss and prostate cancer. They found that men with bald spots at the top of their heads were one and a half times more likely to have prostate cancer than those without bald spots. The association was particularly strong for men who were diagnosed with high-grade prostate cancer at 60–69 years of age."[2]

One cultural myth has been that men with too much testosterone—in other words, men perceived as very virile—are the ones who lose their hair most rapidly, until reaching baldness. The key is not your testosterone levels, but rather the levels of the enzyme which converts testosterone into DHT, the other factor being whether your hair follicles are highly sensitized to DHT.

Destressing (chronic stress can affect hair health) and testosterone replacement may provide some defense against hair thinning and hair loss. There is also evidence supporting taking these steps: Low iron and vitamin D levels contribute to hair thinning and can be remedied with supplements. Herbs that help preserve hair may include saw palmetto and ginkgo biloba.

Also, eat foods rich in iron (kale, spinach) and vitamin C (red pepper, broccoli) and vitamin A (sweet potato, kale) and zinc (chickpeas and mung bean sprouts). Use essential oils like rosemary, spikenard, and peppermint, mixed together and applied to the scalp. Acupuncture has also been shown to have positive effects in stimulating blood flow to the scalp.

Finasteride and Dutasteride as Pharmaceutical Treatments

Scientists first developed a medication called finasteride to treat both baldness and benign prostatic hyperplasia by blocking the conversion of testosterone to DHT. The 5 mg dose version is called Proscar, while a 1 mg dose is sold as Propecia.

Later, other scientists developed dutasteride (also known as Avodart), which works in a similar way as finasteride to block DHT. It also works faster and more effectively than finasteride in stimulating hair growth, according to some research studies, but does so with more sexual dysfunction side effects in some patients. (These side effects reversed once use of the drug stopped.)

A study in the *Journal of the American Academy of Dermatology*, compared the two drugs in 416 men, between twenty-one and forty-five years of age. They received dutasteride, finasteride, or a placebo daily for twenty-four weeks. Their conclusion: "Dutasteride increased target area hair count versus placebo in a dose-dependent fashion and dutasteride 2.5 mg was superior to finasteride at 12 and 24 weeks." Dutasteride produced 109 hairs of new growth compared to 75 hairs for finasteride.[3]

Nearly a decade later, another science team writing in the same medical journal reported, after assessing dutasteride versus finasteride in 917 men, aged twenty to fifty years, that dutasteride "significantly increased hair count and width and improved hair growth at week 24 compared with finasteride and placebo." Also, the scientists concluded, "the number and severity of adverse events (side effects) were similar among treatment groups."[4]

Natural Solution: Red Ginseng Oil

Red ginseng, a type of steamed and dried ginseng, has been a fixture of traditional Asian medicine for thousands of years, and in the past decade received scientific scrutiny as a possible hair loss remedy by applying the oil to the scalp.

In a 2017 study in the science journal *Molecules*, Korean scientists tested it on lab animals and concluded, "Hair regenerative capacity was significantly restored by treatment of red ginseng oil . . . these results suggest that red ginseng oil is a potent novel therapeutic natural product for treatment of androgenic alopecia through hair re-growth activity of its major components."[5]

Previous research, using lab animals, into the safety of red ginseng oil had found it to be "a safe and nontoxic" herbal medicine for humans, with a wide range of therapeutic treatment applications.[6]

Natural Solution: *Schisandra nigra* and *Crinum asiaticum*

Two plants native to Jeju Island, in South Korea, have been extensively studied in lab animal experiments by Korean scientists for their hair growth potential. *Schisandra nigra* was evaluated in the *European Journal of Dermatology* in 2009: "These results suggest that *S. nigra* extract has the potential to promote hair growth."[7] *Crinum asiaticum* was also evaluated in the *European Journal of Dermatology*, with scientists concluding in 2010, "These results suggest that norgalanthamine (a principal ingredient of *C. asisaticum*) has the potential to promote hair growth."[8]

Natural Solution: *Thuja orientalis* and *Eclipta alba*

An East Asia evergreen shrub or small tree, *Thuja orientalis* has been studied in science labs based on its reputation as a traditional cure for baldness or hair loss in Eastern Asian countries. A 2013 study in lab animals concluded, "These results suggest that *T. orientalis* extract promotes hair growth by inducing the anagen phase in resting hair follicles and might therefore be a potential hair growth-promoting agent."[9]

A medicinal plant from the Ayurveda tradition of India, *Eclipta alba* (also known as false daisy) received scientific attention with experiments using lab animals because of the plant's longstanding reputation of promoting hair growth in men. In a 2009 study, published in the *Journal of Ethnopharmacology*, scientists concluded, "These findings suggest that methanol extract of *Eclipta alba* may have potential as a hair growth promoter."[10]

Natural Solution: Dihomo-y-linolenic acid (DGLA)

Italian scientists have been working with several formulations of dihomo-y-linolenic acid (DGLA), which is a precursor of the prostaglandin PGE1, which they have applied as topical lotion for both men and women. It apparently increases microcirculation of the scalp and reduces the toxic action of elevated dihydrotestosterone levels on the hair bulbs.

In a 2018 study, two versions of the lotion were tested on thirty men and thirty women, average age of forty-six for men and forty-nine for women. After six months of treatment, daily topical applications of both lotion variations "resulted in a hair count that significantly increased for women and marginally increased for men."[11]

Overcoming Fatigue 9

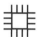

IF YOU'RE EXPERIENCING CHRONIC TIREDNESS and fatigue, it could be due to low testosterone, which in turn can be a trigger for sleep disturbances, or anxiety and depression, which on their own or together can further contribute to your lack of vitality. Being tired all the time, no matter how much caffeine you ingest, may be a sign that you've entered andropause.

It's important to go through a checklist of possible underlying conditions, which could help to explain your tiredness and fatigue, particularly if this state has been persistent and doesn't seem to clear up after prolonged rest or the resolution of any chronic stress you've been under. Going through this checklist may require some diagnostic testing with blood work and physical examination by a trained physician.

1. *Chronic fatigue syndrome*, also known in medical literature as systemic exertion intolerance disease, always has cognitive problems accompanying the fatigue, such as short-term memory deficits and verbal dyslexia. An infectious agent has been hypothesized to be responsible for the condition. Only a physician, using clinical criteria, can diagnose chronic fatigue syndrome.
2. *Anemia* is characterized by fatigue caused by a low red blood cell count, which can be due to an iron deficiency, or a

deficiency in folate and vitamin B-12. Blood testing can determine whether you have this condition.

3. *Hypothyroidism* is caused by the thyroid gland failing to produce enough T3 and T4 hormones. Fatigue is a common symptom, but so is muscle weakness, thinning hair, sensitivity to cold, and depression. If none of these symptoms are present, your fatigue is due to reasons other than your thyroid gland.

4. *Sleep disorders* like obstructive sleep apnea can cause fatigue, but sleepiness, the inability to remain alert or fully awake in the daytime, becomes a distinguishing factor in making a diagnosis.

These four medical conditions are some of the most common factors, outside of the low testosterone factor, causing fatigue. Other possible medical factors to keep in mind as causes—all of which are replete with symptoms other than fatigue—include autoimmune disorders, chronic infections, diabetes, cancer, gastrointestinal disorders, cardiovascular disease, and side effects from some pharmaceutical drugs.

Over-Exercising Triggers Low Testosterone and Chronic Fatigue

We know how resistance training and aerobic exercise can boost testosterone levels in most men, but were you aware there is a tipping point where strenuous exercise can actually result in plummeting testosterone levels and chronic fatigue? A case study of this phenomenon was provided by America's fastest marathoner in 2016, Boston Marathon winner Ryan Hall, who retired from the sport due to chronically low testosterone levels that brought on debilitating fatigue, all due to overtraining.

Scientists had previously documented this condition by noting how endurance athletes "exhibit persistently reduced free and total testosterone concentrations." Though "the exact physiological mechanism inducing the reduction of testosterone in these men is currently unclear," scientists reported in the study, they suspect it is a dysfunction in the interaction between the brain's hypothalamus and the pituitary gland.[1]

In a 2010 study in the *Journal of Sexual Medicine*, 183 male athletes were studied, their exercise habits assessed, and their total and free testosterone measured in blood testing. Severe or mild testosterone deficiency was found in up to 18 percent of the men, with an average age of sixty-one years, and up to 25 percent deficiency in men seventy years of age and older. Basically, the testosterone-boosting benefits of exercise have been canceled out by too much exercise over a period of years.[2]

A Variety of Natural Options

To rejuvenate energy, not only does testosterone need to be stimulated back to normal levels again, but other dietary and supplementation steps may also need to be taken. Natural remedies to promote testosterone production include *Avena sativa*, *Tribulus terrestris*, fenugreek, and tongkat ali.

Other treatment steps involve the cessation of consuming foods that cause fatigue, such as abandoning animal protein in favor of plant proteins, cutting out unhealthy fats, and avoiding sugars. Chronic stress and lack of quality sleep also depletes energy and must be addressed, as we do in this book, by a holistic program.

For the treatment of fatigue and low libido, Siberian ginseng (Eleuthero), a shrub found in parts of far western Russia, China, and Korea, has roots that have been used as a medicinal for thousands of years. Science lab tests document how the use of Siberian ginseng can help keep levels of male androgens high and the prostate gland healthy.

Natural Solution: Melatonin Supplements

Though melatonin, a hormone made by the pineal gland, is generally viewed only as a sleep aid, when it is synthesized into supplement form, it has also received attention in scientific literature as a fatigue fighter.

In a *European Journal of Neurology* study, twenty-nine patients with chronic fatigue syndrome took 5 mg of melatonin orally each day for three months. Levels of reported fatigue were monitored before, during and after treatment with the supplement. The study results were encouraging: after treatment with melatonin "scores for fatigue, concentration, motivation and activity improved significantly."[3]

It's also useful to note that L-tryptophan, a melatonin precursor, might be effective for some people when taken in supplement form.

Natural Solution: Vitamin B12 Supplements

A deficiency in the body's access to, and absorption of, vitamin B12 can produce symptoms of fatigue, particularly in people on standard diets. Up to 70 percent of people lack sufficient B12 and require supplementation.

Red blood cell formation, neurological functions, and DNA synthesis are some of the important roles that B12 plays in the human body. Older adults generally experience reduced levels of stomach acidity with age, a condition that makes it difficult for them to absorb B12 from food alone. An estimated 15 percent of the general population suffers from this condition, which can produce symptoms of fatigue. Other research has revealed that people in younger age groups (twenty-six to forty-nine years, and fifty to sixty-four years) also show B12 deficiencies as a rate "much greater than previously assumed," according to the U.S. National Institutes of Health, Office of Dietary Supplements.

Both oral living botanicals and injected food-based forms of B12 supplementation have been found to be effective in normalizing B12 levels while reducing the severity of fatigue.[4]

Natural Solution: Coenzyme Q10 Supplementation

CoQ-10, or ubiquinone, is a naturally occurring nutrient, necessary for cell energy, which steadily declines in humans with age. It is found in the heart, kidneys, and liver in concentrations sufficient to act as an energy transfer molecule for these organs because they have high rates of metabolism. A wide array of scientific study evidence shows that taking CoQ-10 supplements, such as Lifegive, "play a significant role in boosting the immune system and physical performance," according to a study review in the *Journal of Pharmacy & Bioallied Sciences*. The generally recommended dosage level is 30–90 mg per day.[5]

Natural Solution: *Rhodiola rosea*

The mountain herb known as *Rhodiola rosea*, grown at high altitudes in northern latitudes, has long had a reputation as an ancient medicinal with energy-boosting physical performance benefits. A series of twenty-first-century medical science studies have affirmed these beneficial effects on energy, physical performance, and mental performance. In a 2011 study survey by the journal *Phytomedicine*, scientists examined results from randomized clinical trials and found a pattern of evidence indicating that the herb "may have beneficial effects" and does so with "few reported mild adverse events" (side effects).[6]

Natural Solution: Ashwagandha Supplementation

An herb from India's ancient Ayurvedic medical tradition, it reportedly enhances energy by strengthening the body's response to stress, both physical and mental.

In a review of five clinical human trials conducted on the herb's effectiveness, scientists at SUNY Upstate Medical University in Syracuse, New York, concluded, "*Withania somnifera* [scientific name for ashwagandha] intervention resulted in greater score improvements (significantly in most cases) than placebo in outcomes on anxiety or stress scales."[7]

A study testing the effectiveness of ashwagandha supplementation on cycling athletes found their endurance improved. The test subjects were given 500 mg capsules of aqueous roots of ashwagandha twice daily for eight weeks. Their aerobic capacity was measured using treadmill tests. As the research team concluded, "There was significant improvement in the experimental group in all parameters" of measurement.[8]

Natural Solution: Stay Hydrated

It may sound like such an obvious factor to avoid fatigue, but drinking enough pure water and staying sufficiently hydrated is too often overlooked once fatigue sets in, particularly when it affects those who are not as young as they once were. One of the first signs of fatigue is when your body signals its need for water. It's a subject that's been well studied over the years.

As a *European Journal of Clinical Nutrition* study pointed out, in 2003, even "chronic mild dehydration" is common in some population groups, "especially the elderly and those who participate in physical activity in warm environments." Impairment of cognitive function, alertness, and overall tiredness and complaints of fatigue often accompany failure to regularly receive adequate fluid intake.[9]

The remedy to fatigue should be water, not consuming sports drinks heavy in sugars and caffeine. This was underscored in research that tested the impact of energy drinks on study subjects and their subsequent sleepiness and fatigue. In a study in Britain, ten test subjects drank a well-known energy drink (containing 42 g of sugars and 30 mg of caffeine), which was compared against a water drink, and then underwent reaction time tests. The previous night, their sleep had been restricted to five hours. Results showed that "the energy drink did not counteract sleepiness and led to slower reaction times" eighty minutes after consumption.[10]

Testosterone Replacement Therapy Can Boost Vitality

Three categories of men experiencing serious fatigue as part of their health conditions have been studied for the impact testosterone replacement has on their energy levels—men with cancer, men with obstructive sleep apnea, and mature men with frailty.

Previous studies had shown that testosterone replacement improved quality of life and diminished fatigue in non-cancer patients. To test its usefulness among men with cancer suffering from fatigue, a 2013 study treated thirteen cancer patients with testosterone and sixteen with a placebo for four weeks. The science team concluded,

"Fatigue scores were significantly better in those treated with testosterone by day 72."[11]

Fatigue is a common symptom associated with obstructive sleep apnea patients, so a research team in 2015, experimented with fifteen patients who had been diagnosed with the condition, and fifteen control subjects. Serum testosterone levels and fatigue were compared each day between the two groups. "Among all variables, testosterone was the only independent significant predictor of physical fatigue," the researchers concluded, which they interpreted to mean testosterone replacement therapy was a viable option to diminish fatigue levels.[12]

Finally, among 274 frail men, sixty-five years of age and older, with free testosterone levels at or below 250 pmol/liter, researchers divided them into a transdermal testosterone gel group and a placebo gel group, for six months of testing. The findings were conclusive: "Testosterone treatment in intermediate-frail and frail elderly men with low to borderline-low T for 6 months may prevent age-associated loss of lower limb muscle strength and improve body composition, quality of life [vitality], and physical function."[13]

Managing Chronic Stress 10

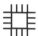

Y OUR HORMONE LEVELS ARE AFFECTED by your sleep quality and your level of chronic stress. One condition reinforces
the other. A chronic release of cortisol, the stress hormone,
undermines testosterone levels.

If you have excess stress going on in your life, it can increase
cortisol or sex hormone–binding globulin (SHBG). This excess cortisol robs the body of the chemical building blocks of testosterone.
In addition, SHBG traps free testosterone, making it unavailable for
use by the body.

To determine the direct impact of job-related stress on male testosterone levels, Japanese scientists recruited 183 men, with an age
range of thirty-four to sixty-seven years, working at a midsize company, and measured their testosterone in blood samples, along with
compiling assessments to profile their job demands, health behaviors,
and history of disease. Those men with the highest psychological job
demands had the most serious testosterone deficiencies and the most
andropause symptoms.[1]

A follow-up study with the same group of Japanese men, conducted four years later, checked to see whether reduced job demands
in the company for some of them had impacted their testosterone
levels. It turned out those men who had experienced reduced job demands, and thus lower stress levels, had increased their testosterone,
as measured in blood tests.[2]

Any stress-reduction regimen probably needs to address how chronic stress suppresses the immune system, literally shrinks the human brain, worsens the effects of toxic chemical exposure, and depletes testosterone in men. Engaging in mindfulness meditation practices and using affirmations both have strong scientific backing for reducing stress. So does receiving daily doses of laughter from humorous movies, TV comedies, and other media.

Natural Solution: Korean *Panax Ginseng*

Numerous science studies have uncovered evidence that the root of *Panax ginseng*, used as a multifaceted medicinal plant in traditional medicine for thousands of years, has an antistress effect on the human body, directly influencing the adrenal glands, which are highly sensitive to stress.[3] The most common types, or families, of ginseng are Siberian, Chinese, and American, each with different active compounds and different effects on the human body.[4]

Korean ginseng, from the Chinese ginseng family, contains thirty-eight ginsenosides (the major active pharmacological components) compared to just nineteen ginsenosides in American ginseng, making the Korean version a more highly sought-after and studied herbal treatment.[5]

Natural Solution: Curcumin Supplementation

Curcumin is a key component of the spice turmeric, which has long been a fixture in both the cuisine and the Ayurvedic medicine tradition of India. Consuming curcumin has been documented to reverse the cellular damage caused by chronic stress and to exert beneficial antidepression effects on the brain.

Here is how the science journal *Critical Reviews in Food Science and Nutrition* described curcumin in 2017: "A type of herb belonging to [the] ginger family, which is widely grown in southern and south western tropical Asia region. Turmeric is known to have been used for centuries in India and China for the medical treatments of such illnesses as dermatologic diseases, infection, stress, and depression.

Curcumin is known recently to have antioxidant, anti-inflammatory, anticancer effects and, thanks to these effects, to have an important role in prevention and treatment of various illnesses."[6]

Scientists at the University of California at Los Angeles investigated the effect of curcumin consumption on brain deficits of DHA, an acid essential to brain function whose deficit is linked to stress and anxiety. Both lab animal tests and test tube testing of curcumin revealed it to be a potent booster of DHA in the brain, resulting in a reduction of stress and anxiety symptoms.[7]

Natural Solution: Therapeutic Laughter

For decades, the international magazine *Reader's Digest* featured a regular column titled "Laughter Is the Best Medicine." It was a truism more accurate than the editors of that publication could have ever suspected. Stress-relieving effects on the mind and body from engaging in therapeutic laughter have come to be studied recently for a variety of ailments, after initial research found laughter to have positive effects on the human immune system.

Laughter almost instantly reduces blood pressure and releases endorphins, nicknamed the body's "feel good" chemicals, while lowering the levels of cortisol, the stress hormone, circulating in the body.

In a 2015 study, scientists exposed thirty-one cancer patients, to a therapeutic laughter program to test the extent to which it could reduce measures of anxiety, depression, and stress. The biggest score reduction from laughter was in the stress category, and that occurred after only one session, prompting the research team to conclude, "It could be recommended as a first-line therapy" for the treatment of stress.[8]

A second study, this one done with ninety-one healthy students, had half assigned to a laughter intervention group and the other half to a control group. Measures were then taken of the diagnostic impact on their bodies after the students were exposed to fifteen minutes of stressful testing. Just hearing laughter, not necessarily participating in it, resulted in significant decreases in stress among the group assigned to the intervention.[9]

Natural Solution: Mindfulness-Based Stress Reduction

A program developed at the University of Massachusetts Medical Center in the 1970s used mindfulness to treat anxiety, stress, and depression with a combination of meditation, deep breathing, present-moment awareness, and a mental state characterized by detachment.

A 2018 study tested a mindfulness-based stress-reduction program on 110 nurses, all in high-stress jobs, who were randomly assigned to either an eight-week intervention or a control group. The study found that "the intervention group showed decreases in stress and negative affect and increases in positive affect and resilience after the intervention."[10]

Another 2018 study, published in the journal *Stress Health*, investigated the effects of the program on infertile women, aged eighteen to fifty years, experiencing chronic stress as a result of their medical condition. Sixty-two women were assigned to the intervention group and thirty-seven women to a control group. After eight weeks, it was found that the intervention group "had reduced stress and depressive symptoms while increasing general well-being."[11]

Natural Solution: A Yoga Practice

Developed several thousand years ago, in India, yoga is a physical movement practice that involves a series of physical poses, called asanas. The practice has long been thought to bestow mental and physical health benefits, including stress reduction and improved immunity.

A systematic review of yoga as a stress reduction method, comparing a multitude of published scientific journal study findings, was conducted in 2017 by the science journal *Psychoneuroendocrinology*. Forty-two clinical trial studies were included in the comparative assessment.

According to the overview of these cumulative results, "Practices that include yoga asanas were associated with reduced evening cortisol, waking cortisol, ambulatory systolic blood pressure, resting heart rate, high-frequency heart rate variability, fasting blood glucose, cholesterol and low density lipoprotein, compared to active control." In other words, improved regulation of the sympathetic nervous system, as happens with a yoga practice, results in stress relief and better managing of stress.[12]

Countering Sleep Decline 11

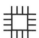

IF YOU REGULARLY EXPERIENCE INSOMNIA, it can be due to having a low level of testosterone. Because growth hormone is produced during sleep as well, disturbances of your natural sleep rhythms can deplete this hormone, adding to the impact already being caused by age-induced andropause.

Both testosterone and growth hormone are released according to a man's circadian rhythm. If he sacrifices deep sleep, which regulates circadian rhythm, he depletes the body's reserves of testosterone. One indicator might be if your memory and judgment seem to be impaired more than normal, and you no longer feel like you have the vitality and energy you need to get through each day. Deep sleep keeps that rhythm in balance, but if you sacrifice sleep, you are inadvertently sacrificing testosterone.

You need to also rule out whether you have a sleep disorder, rather than a testosterone or growth hormone deficiency, to determine why you are chronically sleep deprived. Sleep apnea is one such disorder, in which breathing stops and then starts again throughout the night. Another, more serious variation is *obstructive sleep apnea*, in which loud snoring typically accompanies the breathing interruptions. Still another sleep interruption condition to be watchful of is called *circadian rhythm disorder*, when aging lowers the body's levels of melatonin, disrupting the body's internal sleep clock.

If you suspect you have a sleep disorder, find a physician who specializes in sleep treatments, because, if left untreated, this can become a health impairment leading to a weakened immune system, memory problems, accelerated aging, and an increased risk for strokes and heart attacks.[1]

Numerous scientific studies have documented the link between sleep disruption and low testosterone. Israeli scientists compared a group of healthy middle-aged men to a group of healthy young men, measuring their testosterone levels during sleep. They found significant differences in how much testosterone middle-aged men secrete at night (it is much less than young men), particularly when a disconnect occurs between REM (rapid eye movement) sleep and nighttime testosterone secretion.[2]

This same Israeli science group, in a separate experiment, documented how getting fragmented sleep at night disrupts a man's testosterone secretion rhythm. Their findings opened up subsequent new avenues of research by other science teams, investigating the usefulness of testosterone replacement therapy as part of a treatment regimen for sleep disorders like sleep apnea.[3]

Many evidence-based antidotes exist to treat sleep deprivation based on natural, non-drug treatments. These range from acupuncture (which has dozens of studies supporting its efficacy) to autogenic training, biofeedback, cognitive behavioral therapy, dietary changes (eating tart cherries before bedtime boosts natural melatonin), guided imagery, mindfulness meditation, and other breathing and relaxation techniques.

Let's start with testosterone replacement using bioidentical hormones.

Natural Solution: Testosterone Replacement Therapy

Much of the testosterone research regarding sleep has centered on treating sleep apnea and its more serious offshoot, obstructive sleep apnea. A review of the study literature by physicians at the Mount Sinai School of Medicine, in 2016, concluded that obstructive sleep apnea, which contributes to fatigue and sexual dysfunction among middle-aged men, can have these and other symptoms effectively treated by testosterone replacement. There is evidence that testosterone replacement "alters ventilatory responses" in those with the sleep disorder to lessen its symptoms.[4]

A 2019 study, published in the *World Journal of Men's Health*, affirmed the usefulness of testosterone replacement therapy in treating obstructive sleep apnea (OSA) but cautioned the replacement "may exacerbate OSA in some patients," primarily in patients with severe untreated OSA, so patients interested in starting the treatment should confer with medical specialists.[5]

Finally, a 2017 study from Russia examined twenty-six men, average age of forty-six years, who had both low testosterone and obstructive sleep apnea, and examined the effect on them of a combined treatment of testosterone replacement (using Androgel) and a device called continuous positive airway pressure. Not only did total testosterone levels double over the two-month study period, but a correction of the sleep obstruction also occurred that improved quality of life.[6]

Natural Solution: Melatonin Supplementation

Most pharmaceutical remedies for insomnia and sleep disorders— benzodiazepines, antidepressants, antihistamines, and anxiolytics— carry with them side effects and the potential for dependence and addiction, so that makes natural alternative treatments options that are well worth looking into.

Melatonin, a hormone produced by the pineal gland and released exclusively at night, is the human body's natural regulator of sleep patterns and its diminishment with age can trigger insomnia and other sleep disturbances. In a review of the scientific literature on using melatonin supplementation, the journal *Neurology Research*, in 2017, found it to be an effective "alternative treatment to the currently available pharmaceutical therapies for sleep disorders with significantly less side effects."

Its specific advantages, reported the science team that did the assessments, is that melatonin "has been shown to synchronize the circadian rhythms, and improve the onset, duration and quality of sleep."[7]

Natural Solution: An Amino Acid Preparation

A combination of two amino acid formulations may spell insomnia relief for some sleep disorder patients.

L-tryptophan is an amino acid used to treat insomnia and anxiety; a chemical byproduct from it is 5-HTP, which is produced commercially from the seeds of an African plant called *Griffonia simplicifolia*. Sleep disorder treatment with 5-HTP works on the brain by increasing its production of serotonin, a hormone that affects sleep.

A commercial amino acid formula called Gabadone, in combination with 5-HTP, has been tested for its combined impact on sleep duration and sleep quality. In a study with eighteen sleep disorder patients, half were assigned to either a treatment group or a placebo control group, and they were monitored using diagnostic tests.

In the amino acid treatment group, the baseline time to fall asleep fell from thirty-two minutes to nineteen minutes after treatment, compared to no change in the control group. Nearly two more hours of quality sleep were added each night among treatment patients, compared to no appreciable change in sleep duration in the control group.

"The difference between the active and placebo groups was significant," commented the study authors. "Ease of falling asleep, awakenings, and morning grogginess improved" in the treatment group, as did "increased duration of sleep, and improved quality of sleep."[8]

Natural Solution: Tart Cherry Consumption

Most of us know how certain foods can disrupt sleep as a result of heartburn or acid reflux. Some of the triggers are spicy foods and anything with caffeine or the amino acid tyrosine in it.

What aren't as widely publicized are foods or juices with the power to induce sleepiness or to deepen sleep. One of those evidence-backed insomnia remedies is tart cherry juice.

Research has shown that ingesting tart cherry juice a few hours before bedtime enhances the body's melatonin production, the body's own natural sleep aid. In a *European Journal of Nutrition* study, twenty persons ingested tart cherry juice over seven days and recorded their sleep quality and sleep duration. Periodic urine sampling was done to measure melatonin.

The study findings were so promising that the nutrition scientists recommended anyone with insomnia should drink two glasses of the juice each day to get a better night's rest.[9]

Natural Solution: Acupuncture

Acupuncture is an ancient practice developed in China that uses slender needles applied to specific trigger points in the body. It has achieved scientific legitimacy over the past few decades in several realms of health condition research.

In a systematic review of results from forty-six scientific studies of acupuncture's use in treating insomnia, scientists in 2009 concluded, "Acupuncture appears to be effective in treatment of insomnia. Acupuncture was shown to be superior to medications in lengthening sleep duration by up to three hours. There were no documented side effects from the use of acupuncture, whereas the sleep medications all had some side effects."[10]

Another technique related to acupuncture with needles, and based on the same principles, is acupressure, which relies on applying fingers to pressure points. It has also been studied in relationship to sleep treatment. A study published in the *Journal of Gerontology & Biological Sciences* experimented with pressure point application on eighty-four senior citizens who had insomnia and other sleep disturbances. The findings were clear: "This study confirmed the effectiveness of acupressure in improving the quality of sleep of elderly people and offered a nonpharmacological therapy method for sleep-disturbed mature people."[11]

Natural Solution: Autogenic Training

This relaxation technique was designed to lower blood pressure and calm the mind and body. It involves six simple exercises, done while reclining or sitting, accompanied by a visual imagery technique.

The technique has been studied as a natural alternative to pharmaceutical drugs to treat insomnia. It has no side effects, unlike sleep drugs.

In a British study, 153 patients associated with a sleep disorder clinic did the training daily for eight weeks. At completion of the study, researchers found the participants went to sleep faster at night, slept longer, felt they were more rested upon waking, and experienced less overall stress and anxiety in their life.[12]

Natural Solution: Cognitive Behavioral Therapy

This evidence-based technique needs to be done with a trained therapist, who acts as both teacher and facilitator, to demonstrate to the patient how to substitute positive thoughts for negative thoughts as a way of clearing the mind when recurrent thoughts cause insomnia.

The nonprofit National Sleep Foundation describes how the technique works for insomnia:

> Cognitive Behavioral Therapy for Insomnia, often called CBT-1, is an approved method for treating insomnia without the use of sleeping pills. Sounds impossible? It isn't. Sounds like hard work? It can be. CBT is aimed at changing sleep habits and scheduling factors, as well as misconceptions about sleep and insomnia, that perpetuate sleep difficulties. In fact, the recent National Institute of Health state-of-the-science meeting on insomnia concluded that CBT-1 is a safe and effective means of managing chronic insomnia and its effects. Cognitive behavioral therapy for insomnia includes regular, often weekly, visits to a clinician, who will give you a series of sleep assessments, ask you to complete a sleep diary and work with you in sessions to help you change the way you sleep.[13]

In a 2015 study review, appearing in the *Annals of Internal Medicine*, the findings of twenty studies on sleep and cognitive behavioral therapy were compared to determine the extent to which the findings were similar. All of the studies found positive impacts for the technique on sleep quality. The reviewers wrote, "Cognitive Behavioral Therapy is an effective treatment for adults with chronic insomnia."[14]

Natural Solution: Guided Imagery

Imagination can be a key component to quieting the mind and easing the transition into restful sleep. The technique that has been widely studied for harnessing the imagination to treat insomnia is *guided imagery*, the visualization of a serene forest or water scene, or whatever else the insomniac finds most calming.

An experiment out of Britain's Oxford University illustrates one such study with a positive treatment outcome. Test subjects were forty-one people with chronic insomnia who were given a guided imagery procedure to practice before attempting to fall asleep. The research team called it "imagery distraction," and it showed an almost universal success rate at enabling the test subjects to fall asleep faster and sleep more soundly.

"The success of the imagery distraction task is attributed to it occupying sufficient 'cognitive space' to keep the individual from re-engaging with thoughts, worries, and concerns during the pre-sleep period," the research team concluded.[15]

Natural Solution: Mindfulness Meditation

Sit in a relaxed posture, eyes closed, focus your awareness on your breath, and when your attention wanders (and it will), bring your attention back to your slow, in-and-out breathing through the nostrils. Try to sit still, doing this for ten to twenty minutes each session, each day. That is the essence of the practice of mindfulness meditation.

This relaxation technique, based on the twenty-five-hundred-year-old Buddhist practice called Vipassana meditation, has seen its health benefits studied intensively over the past few decades since its introduction in the United States for stress relief in the 1970s.

One of these studies, published in the *Journal of the American Medical Association's Internal Medicine*, in 2015, examined fifty persons with an average age of sixty-six years who reported insomnia. They were divided into two study groups. The first group did a daily, six-week meditation program; the other group only took classroom instruction on how to maintain good sleep habits.

The research team reported in their science journal article how their study results demonstrated "significant improvement" in the sleep duration and sleep quality of the test subjects, compared to the control group who only received classroom instruction. Less anxiety and stress overall was also a positive outcome for the meditation group.[16]

Natural Solution: The Relaxation Response

Still another relaxation technique with science backing for its effectiveness is called the Relaxation Response. It was developed by Herbert Benson, a Harvard Medical School professor, experimenting with a self-help approach to treating anxiety, stress, and insomnia.

A review of the technique, done at the University of California at Davis, gives a step-by-step explanation for how to perform it, while describing the science behind its effectiveness. Since insomnia is a first sign of stress, the key factor in how the relaxation technique works is its relief of that underlying stress, which is a culprit in producing the worrisome thoughts that trigger or contribute to the symptoms of insomnia.[17]

After reviewing the findings of several hundred studies on the Relaxation Response, the *Journal of Alternative and Complementary Medicine* concluded it was a safe and effective antidote to insomnia and works for most people who make it a regular regimen for their life.[18]

Natural Solution: Napping

It may sound deceptively simple: you just lie down in the afternoon and sleep for a few minutes to rejuvenate your mind and body. However, there is more napping it than that, and science research has affirmed its usefulness if you have the time and patience to integrate naps into your daily routine.

In a review of the science appearing in the *Journal of Sleep Research*, dozens of napping studies were evaluated and their findings compared. Studies were found showing that combining a thirty-minute afternoon nap with moderate intensity exercise in the evening improved all measures of sleep quality at night.

Universally, study results indicated that older adults get as much benefit from short naps as young people; napping leads to improvements in cognitive performance in all age groups; stress is relieved; and the nap and exercise combination improved daytime alertness, concentration, strength, and coordination. Moods and overall well-being also improved after napping.[19]

Stopping Breast Growth   12

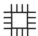

A T LEAST TWICE IN THE AVERAGE male's life he will grow
identifiable breasts—for a small period of time in childhood,
and for a much longer period, perhaps for life, in adulthood,
usually starting in his fifties or sixties. Both periods in a man's life—
puberty and later life—are when a cyclic imbalance of the hormones
testosterone and estrogen occurs (testosterone decreases, estrogen
increases), creating a condition called gynecomastia, a swelling of
breast tissue.

Up to 70 percent of all men will grow breast tissue by the age of
sixty-nine years, according to the Mayo Clinic, and it can cause some
men considerable male image anxiety, particularly if their breasts
begin to resemble that of a small-breasted woman. If it occurs as a
result of non-hormonal overall weight gain, physicians tend to call
it chest flab, but just as often the growth is a byproduct of the drop
in testosterone that occurs with andropause.[1] As breast tissue grows,
so does the risk for male breast cancer, though the incidence of this
cancer in men is low, just 1 percent of all cases reported.[2]

Other Causes of Breast Growth
Hops in beer can be a breast enlarger that also causes prostate inflammation and helps trigger BPH (benign prostatic hyperplasia). Hops
are a testosterone antagonist because the hop plant is powerfully

estrogenic, containing estradiol, which, once consumed by a male, lowers testosterone. Breast growth is particularly pronounced in male chronic abusers of alcohol, but in recent decades it has become more common in men who consume hoppy beer, especially the IPA craft-beer type.[3]

As discussed earlier in this book, *marijuana is an androgen hormone antagonist*. Some of the chemicals found in the marijuana plant disrupt a man's androgen hormones, while having estrogen-like effects on the male body, an imbalance that can result in the growth of breast tissue in some susceptible men.[4]

There can also be *environmental causes*. For example, an epidemic of gynecomastia occurred among young Haitian male refugees in U.S. detention centers during the 1980s. New onset breast growth appeared suddenly in twenty out of every two hundred or so men screened once they were living in the centers. A subsequent investigation found a chemical component of a delousing spray applied to bedding was the androgen antagonist culprit. Most of the breast growth symptoms went away once the lice-killing agent was discontinued.[5]

There can also be *food consumption causes*. A diet high in estrogen-laden foods can trigger breast growth in some men. Such a case was profiled in a science journal in 2008. A sixty-year-old man began experiencing unexplained breast growth accompanied by erectile dysfunction and decreased libido. All diagnostic testing revealed everything to be normal. Subsequent investigation revealed that he was drinking three quarts of soy milk every day. After he discontinued soy consumption, his estradiol concentrations and breast size slowly returned to normal.[6]

Some herbal products can also induce breast tissue growth in men. "Plant oils, such as tea tree or lavender, used in shampoos, soaps or lotions have been associated with gynecomastia. This is probably due to their weak estrogenic activity," reported the Mayo Clinic.[7]

There can be breast growth related to a man's treatment for prostate cancer. Hormonal therapy can create "a significant problem in men" with breast growth, according to a 2005 study in the *Journal of Urology*. "In large, randomized, placebo-controlled studies approximately 50 percent or more of patients with prostate cancer experienced gynecomastia due to multiple mechanisms," the Johns Hopkins

University School of Medicine research team reported. "Although its severity was mostly reported as mild to moderate, gynecomastia was cited as the reason for most premature withdrawals from therapy." As a treatment, these study authors recommended tamoxifen.[8] Observing the overall effects of tamoxifen in our decades of work leads us to encourage an alternative.

Mainstream Medicine Remedies for Male Breast Growth

Tamoxifen—one of the oldest of hormone therapies, blocks the effects of estrogen in breast tissue, as part of a cancer treatment and prevention regimen for women. It has also been used in men for breast cancer and to reduce breast swelling.

In a 2018 study of tamoxifen therapy for gynecomastia, scientists from Oxford University and the University of Cambridge did ten years of observation of eighty-one patients with an average age of forty-two years when the study began, who took 10 mg daily. The scientists concluded, "Our results show approximately nine in every 10 men treated with tamoxifen therapy had successful resolution of their symptoms."[9]

Liposuction—"If the gynecomastia is entirely due to fat, suction lipectomy alone is sufficient treatment," observed the science journal *Plastic Reconstructive Surgery* after evaluating the use of liposuction since 1980, the year it became the cornerstone of treatment for male breast enlargement.[10]

Breast Reduction Surgery—A radical though minimally invasive surgical technique, it involves using traditional liposuction in conjunction with a shaver that removes the fibrofatty and glandular tissues of the male breast. A study of twenty-five patients given this procedure showed it was effective and provided consistent results.[11]

Natural Solution: Weight Loss

It's well documented that visceral fat causes inflammation and insulin resistance, and that can decrease testosterone production. This excess body fat can cause the testosterone that is available in the body to convert to estrogen, which results in the development of male breasts. That alone should be reason enough for any man undergoing andropause to want those excess pounds to melt away from his waistline, not to mention all of the other health benefits that can be achieved from losing weight.

It is important to combine a weight-loss regimen of exercise and dietary change with a conscious eye toward boosting testosterone production in the body. One place to start on the dietary front is consuming high-fiber vegetables, which helps to remove excess estrogen that is contributing to breast growth. Among the highest-fiber vegetables are acorn squash, artichokes, broccoli, chia seeds, collard greens, green peas, navy beans, spinach, sweet potatoes, Swiss chard, pea sprouts, and sunflower sprouts.

Coupled with dietary intervention, as part of an exercise regimen, chest tightening exercises might be recommended for some men as part of a resistance-training routine for optimal testosterone production.

For more on weight-loss strategies, see the next chapter of this book.

Reversing Weight Gain 13

B Y NOW, IN READING THIS BOOK, you're probably getting a sense of how interconnected male hormone imbalances can be to all of the many symptoms of andropause and that they most often occur together. As a man puts on extra pounds, his testosterone is converted into estrogen. That further reduces his testicles' ability to produce more testosterone. This cycle is exacerbated by age-related andropause, which further lowers testosterone, producing even more fat retention.

Attracting visceral fat around the midsection causes inflammation and insulin resistance; that, in turn, further decreases testosterone production. Having excessive body fat can convert remaining testosterone to estrogen, leading to the development of those unsightly flaps of man breasts, as discussed in the previous chapter.

There is scientific evidence supporting these entanglements: "Obesity is associated with a reduction of serum testosterone and, vice versa, a reduction in serum testosterone is associated with obesity and features of the metabolic syndrome," commented a 2014 report in the journal *Obesity Research & Clinical Practice*.[1]

These connections are a big ball of thorny twine and present a challenge for any normal person to untangle. What is needed is a holistic treatment approach. It all begins with a focus on reducing weight to a number within the normal range for a given age and height.

One research team writing in the *European Journal of Endocrinology* put the challenge in stark terms after examining 2,736 men, aged forty to seventy-nine years: "Weight loss was associated with a rise [in testosterone], free testosterone, and sex hormone–binding globulin. Weight management appears to be important in maintaining circulating testosterone in ageing men, and obesity-associated changes in the hypothalamic-pituitary-testicular axis hormones are reversible following weight reduction."[2]

Increasing Your Risk for Metabolic Syndrome

A sort of worst-case scenario, albeit a common one, for weight gain and testosterone loss is the appearance of a cluster of conditions that medical science refers to as metabolic syndrome. This is characterized by excess body fat around the waist, high blood pressure, abnormal cholesterol, and triglyceride levels, which together greatly increase risk of diabetes, stroke, and heart disease.

A large team of scientists, describing their 2015 study, published in the *Journal of Clinical Endocrinology Metabolism*, noted how low testosterone, by itself, can be an independent trigger for developing metabolic syndrome. They evaluated 3,369 men, aged forty to seventy-nine years, and identified those who diagnostic testing showed were at risk for the health syndrome. The trend was borne out so clearly that the scientists declared, "Men with lower baseline [start of the study] total testosterone levels were at higher risk for developing [metabolic syndrome]."[3]

If you're overweight with low testosterone and you don't exercise enough, you're writing yourself a ticket to metabolic syndrome and an unhealthy, shorter life. The antidote to this condition sounds easier on paper than it may be in practice for most men—just lose the excess weight. Read on to learn some tips for success!

The Hidden Role of Obesogens in Weight Gain

Obesogens are endocrine disrupter chemicals from food, food packaging, personal care products, pesticides, and the environment that act on the human body in such a way as to induce obesity by disrupting normal fat metabolism. Combined with an unhealthy diet and a lack of aerobic exercise, these become the "unholy trinity" of triggers for excess weight—and worse, for obesity and the virtual extermination of testosterone from the male body.

These chemical toxins are stored in the body's fat cells, especially in the visceral fat that collects around the abdomen. Nutritional deficiencies, the lack of enough "scavenger" anti-inflammatory nutrients in the body, compound the problem by failing to eliminate these toxins from fat cells fast enough. The world's largest organization of hormone specialists, the Endocrine Society, has declared over the past decade, "The rise in the incidence in obesity matches the rise in the use and distribution of industrial chemicals that may be playing a role in a generation of obesity, suggesting Endocrine Disrupting Chemicals (EDCs) may be linked to this epidemic."[4]

This connection may be a key reason why there are currently more obese humans on the planet than underweight humans, irrespective of age. According to *The Lancet*, a British medical journal, which compiled worldwide health statistics from 1975 to 2014, this was a period when global obesity in men tripled, and obesity in women more than doubled.[5]

"The increasing incidence of obesity is a serious global public health challenge," declared scientists with the U.S. National Institute of Environmental Health Sciences, a division of the National Institutes of Health. "Although the obesity epidemic is largely fueled by poor nutrition and lack of exercise, certain chemicals have been shown to potentially have a role. These chemicals, so-called 'obesogens' might predispose some individuals to gain weight despite their efforts to limit caloric intake and increase levels of physical activity."[6]

According to several studies examining obesogens in the U.S. food supply, "food is the major route of exposure to endocrine disrupters," reported the *Journal of Cancer Prevention*, in 2015. One study took thirty-two food samples from three major supermarket chains in the area around Dallas, Texas, and found high levels of contamination with PBDEs, a toxic endocrine disrupter chemical used as a flame retardant in many consumer products. These residues appeared mainly in fish, meat, and dairy products. PBDEs are known to block the production of testosterone in men.[7]

As we wrote earlier in this book, using a far infrared sauna is one method for purging these toxins from body fat. In a study examining BPA (Bisphenol A), a hormone-disrupting chemical found in plastic food containers, assessing its impact on the human body, scientists in 2012 determined that sweating was an effective way to leach the chemical from the human body. BPA leaches from the lining of beverage and food cans to enter what consumers drink or eat, making it difficult to avoid if you are a consumer of canned food of any sort.[8]

Mainstream Medicine Solution: Bariatric Surgery

One option for drastic weight loss, one that we don't recommend but mainstream medicine does, is bariatric surgery, which restricts the amount of food the human stomach can hold. The most common of these surgeries are gastric band, gastric sleeve, and gastric bypass. Each carries with it a set of risks that need to be investigated before undertaking such an extreme measure. Side effects may include bleeding, infection, internal leakage, and blood clots.[9]

It is worth noting, however, that study assessments of patients following the procedure have found substantial weight loss. About half of adults surveyed had lost up to ninety pounds within three years after the gastric bypass surgery, about one-third of their starting weight. Among gastric band patients, half had lost at least forty-four pounds within three years of undergoing that procedure.[10]

Other studies have found that some men who have undergone bariatric surgery increase their levels of free and total testosterone in the aftermath. In the *European Journal of Endocrinology*, for instance, scientists analyzed twenty-two studies with bariatric surgery findings and saw consistent results pointing to a large increase in testosterone, along with a decrease in estradiol. The more weight male patients lost, the greater the increase in their testosterone afterward.[11]

Mainstream Medicine Solution: Pharmaceutical Drugs

Numerous antiobesity drugs have been developed by the pharmaceutical industry since the late 1990s.

Here is how a review of the evidence for these drugs, published by the European Society of Endocrinology, described their effects in 2015:

> Medical interventions, with the exception of bariatric surgery, have shown limited success, in particular as far as pharmacological treatments are concerned.
>
> Numerous anti-obesity drugs have been developed in the last twenty years, but they have often been suspended from the market because of poor efficacy and /or insufficient safety. The ideal pharmacological intervention should provide a prompt (during the first month) and sustained weight loss after 3-6 months without significant adverse effects. This is a difficult goal to achieve because energy balance regulation is redundant and overlaps with the regulation of other vital systems.[12]

Natural Solution: Supplements and Diet for Metabolic Syndrome

Science research indicates that deficiencies in vitamin D and magnesium have a causal relationship with metabolic syndrome, that cluster of symptoms that is estimated to affect and endanger up to half of all adults in the world at some point in their lives.

In 2018, scientists examined 463 women, aged forty-five to seventy-five years, and tested their vitamin D levels and whether they showed symptoms of metabolic syndrome. They found solid evidence that a deficiency "was associated with a higher prevalence of metabolic syndrome."[13]

Another 2018 study, this one including both men and women between the ages of forty-five and sixty-five years, also uncovered a link between a vitamin D deficiency and abdominal obesity. The more belly fat you have, the lower your vitamin D levels turn out to be, making a case for supplementation after undergoing blood testing to measure vitamin D concentrations.[14]

Concerning the impact of a magnesium deficiency, a study review conducted for the journal *Diabetes Medicine* examined the results of six studies, with 24,473 test subjects, and found a direct link between magnesium deficiency and the prevalence of metabolic syndrome. "For every 100-mg/day increment in magnesium intake," the journal observed, "the overall risk of having metabolic syndrome was lowered by 17%." The authors of this review went on to state that "dietary magnesium intake has been inadequate in the general population in both the USA and worldwide."[15]

Several dietary strategies whose foods are high in both magnesium and vitamin D have also been identified in science research as diets being beneficial to preventing and reversing metabolic syndrome. A study review in the *International Journal of Molecular Science* in 2016 sifted through the evidence supporting specific diets for the prevention and treatment of the cluster of metabolic syndrome symptoms. Three treatments were seen as offering the most verifiable and persuasive results: energy-restricted diets, diets rich in omega-3 fatty acids, and the Mediterranean diet.

The largest body of consistent study evidence supports adherence to a plant-based diet for both weight loss and metabolic syndrome treatment. It's a diet high in fiber intake, antioxidants, and anti-inflammatory nutrients, from its emphasis on plant foods. "Different studies suggest the MedDiet as a successful tool for the prevention and treatment of MetS [metabolic syndrome] and related comorbidities," concluded the study review. "Different studies also suggest that the MedDiet pattern may be a good strategy for obesity treatment as it has been associated with significant reductions in body weight and waist circumference."[16]

Natural Solution: Diets to Lower Weight, Elevate Testosterone

Keep in mind that an estimated one-third of the world's men qualify as overweight or obese as these words are being written, with many millions more candidates for weight gain appearing in the near future, based on demographic trends. Therefore, the information here should be considered useful to just about every man on the planet.[17]

Our first advice, as a huge volume of scientific evidence supports us in saying, is to cut out all junk food of any sort and adopt a plant-based diet. Cut out the dietary sugar and carbohydrates, because the more of that you eat, the more likely it is that you'll develop insulin resistance or diabetes, conditions that exacerbate weight gain and further lower testosterone levels in your body. It's no coincidence that most men with type 2 diabetes are overweight and also have low testosterone.

Our survey of the scientific literature reveals several trends in the findings.

Calorie-Restrictive Diets—Scientists have explored the testosterone-raising impact of diets that restrict the number of calories consumed in a day. This can involve prolonged fasting, alternate day fasts, or simply managing daily food intake to achieve a restriction of calories consumed.

A 2014 study, for example, placed a group of obese men on an 800 kcal/day diet for twelve weeks. Not only did the men lose dozens of pounds, but "caloric restriction significantly increased total testosterone," the study team found. They identified the mechanisms involved as "improvement of testicular function" from the caloric restriction and weight loss, and "reduced conversion of testosterone to estradiol."[18]

High Total Antioxidant Diets—Diets with a high content of spices, herbs, fruits, vegetables, and nuts are associated in science studies with a decreased risk of oxidative stress-related diseases, including obesity. The reason has to do with the natural antioxidants found in these foods, which act as scavengers of free radicals in the body. At a minimum, a consumption of 400 grams a day of high total antioxidants is needed to help lose weight and prevent weight gain.[19]

At our Hippocrates Weight Loss Academy, where we use an organic plant-based diet, we have documented how women on average lose eighteen pounds during our twenty-one-day program, and men lose an average of twenty-two pounds.

Natural Solution: Herbs That Assist Weight Loss

Korean red ginseng (*Panax ginseng*) is one of the more extensively studied medicinal herbs from the ancient Chinese medicine tradition, credited by scientific studies with being useful in preventing and treating diabetes, cardiovascular disease, and a host of other ailments. We can now add obesity to that long list.

Animal studies done in 2017 and 2018 produced compelling evidence that parts of the ginseng root containing saponins, an antioxidative and anti-inflammatory natural chemical, exert anti-obesity effects. The 2017 study, published in the science journal *Nutrients*, tested extracts of both green-leaf and dried-leaf ginseng on obese lab animals and found "a significant decreased body weight," prompting the scientists to declare that "to our knowledge, these findings are the first evidence for the anti-obesity effects of the leaf extracts of Korean ginseng in vivo."[20] Scientists writing in the *Journal of Ethnopharmacology* a year later described having tested ginseng extract on other obese lab animals. They concluded that their findings "demonstrate that ginseng can inhibit obesity," and their results "indicate that ginseng may act like testosterone" in the body to help prevent obesity from occurring in the first place.[21]

While these results need to be replicated in clinical trials among human subjects, these initial findings make ginseng a potential useful and safe treatment for weight reduction and testosterone restoration.

Natural Solution: Testosterone Replacement Therapy

One proven by-product of testosterone replacement therapy is a boost to metabolism, which helps the body to shed extra unwanted pounds. There are many other benefits identified in the large body of scientific research done on testosterone and weight. For example, long-term treatment with testosterone results in sustained weight loss, which can be an antidote to yo-yo dieting and how that puts weight back on within short periods of time.

A 2016 study in the *International Journal of Obesity* examined the effects of testosterone replacement over an eight-year period, in 411 obese men. All men received injections of testosterone undecanoate in three-month intervals. "In all three classes of obesity," the study authors reported, "testosterone therapy produced significant weight loss, decrease in waist circumference and body mass index. . . . [It] appears to be an effective approach to achieve sustained weight loss in obese hypogonadal men irrespective of severity of obesity. Based on these findings we suggest that testosterone therapy offers safe and effective treatment strategy of obesity in hypogonadal men."[22]

Another reason why testosterone replacement therapy is effective for weight loss was identified in 2012, in the journal *Current Diabetes Review.* The study found that testosterone treatment improves mood and energy and reduces fatigue. Thus, it "may motivate men to adhere to diet and exercise regimens designed to combat obesity."[23]

After surveying the overall body of scientific literature on testosterone replacement therapy as an obesity treatment, a scientist at the Boston University School of Medicine wrote a study review in 2014, declaring, "The implication of testosterone therapy in management of obesity in men with testosterone deficiency is of paramount clinical significance, as it produces sustained weight loss without recidivism. These findings represent strong foundations for testosterone therapy in obese men with testosterone deficiency."[24]

For overweight men who have developed metabolic syndrome, it's worth noting another study done at the Boston University School of Medicine, involving 255 men, aged thirty-three to sixty-nine years, where they were given testosterone undecanoate treatments (1,000 mg of Nebido) every twelve weeks for five years.

At the conclusion of the study, there were "marked reductions in systolic and diastolic blood pressure, blood glucose, C-reactive protein," and other positive changes, in addition to the restoration of testosterone levels that produced reductions in total cholesterol, low-density lipoprotein cholesterol, and triglycerides. The study team concluded that long-term testosterone therapy, at physiological levels, ameliorates metabolic syndrome components. T therapy in hypogonadal men thus may help reduce the risk of cardiometabolic diseases.[25]

Treating Prostate Problems   **14**

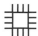

ANDROPAUSE CONTRIBUTES TO prostate enlargement, which in turn, produces an increased urge and frequency to urinate, particularly at night, disrupting sleep quality, a condition that further lowers testosterone production. Once again, we have the "vicious cycle" phenomenon in action.

As testosterone levels are declining, men's estrogen hormones are increasing, by as much as 50 percent, and that in turn, helps the prostate gland to enlarge and trigger *benign prostatic hyperplasia (BPH)*. As a man gains weight, particularly in his midsection, having more fat means testosterone is more quickly converted to estrogen, and as we discussed in a previous chapter, a negative cycle ensues, with prostate health serving as a continuous red flag warning of more potential trouble ahead.

We've already described in this book how hops in beer can enlarge a man's breasts, but it's also important to note that because the hop is a powerful estrogenic plant, containing estradiol, it can cause prostate inflammation and it helps to trigger BPH. There should probably be a warning label about these largely unknown effects pasted on every bottle or can of beer.

BPH can be defined as a mostly age-related condition in which the prostate gland enlarges to cause urinary symptoms, the most common being the partial blockage of urine flow from the bladder. The Mayo Clinic identifies a list of symptoms that men with BPH experience all or most of: frequent or urgent need to urinate, increased frequency at night, difficulty starting a urination stream, a weak start and stop of urine stream, and dribbling at the end of urination.[1]

Here is another prostate condition to be vigilant about—prostatitis.

Prostatitis is a bacterial infection of the prostate causing swelling and inflammation, often triggered when bacteria in the urine leaks into the prostate. The most common symptoms of prostatitis are a frequent urge to urinate (especially at night), an urgent need to urinate, and difficulty urinating. Antibiotics and proven natural remedies are used for this infection, though even one bout with prostatitis may increase a man's chances of initiating a chronic condition.[2]

Mainstream medicine practitioners often prescribe a drug called finasteride for an enlarged prostate, even though a side effect in some men is that it can cause breast enlargement and a decreased libido.

One connection some science studies have drawn is between zinc levels in the prostate and the development of prostatitis. A 2015 review of published studies, for instance, found that "the zinc concentrations in prostatic fluid and seminal plasma from chronic prostatitis patients were significantly lower than normal." Further research was recommended to help determine (the classic "chicken or egg" quandary) whether prostatitis reduces zinc concentrations in the prostate or if a zinc deficiency contributes to prostatitis.[3]

Natural Solution: Zinc Supplementation?

Zinc is important to overall human health, especially to cell regeneration, immune system function, and wound healing, and it plays a direct role in prostate health, where it supports normal sexual functioning of that organ. Though zinc is stored at high levels in the prostate, at levels ten times higher than other soft tissues, it still must constantly be replenished in the body through diet or supplements. For the average adult man, the recommended intake is eleven milligrams a day.

Because we discourage the consumption of animal products and seafood (read our many books on these subjects), which are a common source of zinc, we recommend instead that you draw upon these plant-based dietary sources to get sufficient zinc into your diet:

Beans—chickpeas, lentils, and so on
Nuts—the entire range (excluding peanuts and cashews)
Seeds—pumpkin and hemp seeds in particular
Vegetables—asparagus, kale, mushrooms, peas

There is some evidence that zinc supplementation can help to treat the symptoms of BPH. A 2017 study, for instance, done with seventy-one patients in Italy, had them take a combination of daidzein (a phytoestrogen from beans) and zinc (one tablet a day) for six months, to treat lower urinary symptoms from BPH. The urological study team explained that "in this study, we documented that a combination of daidzein with isolase and zinc, reduces the clinical symptoms of lower urinary tract and improves the quality of life in patients with BPH."[4]

Can Zinc Supplementation Elevate Testosterone?

Zinc is a hormone balancer particularly helpful to testosterone production and maintenance. When a zinc deficiency occurs, "it has a negative effect on serum testosterone concentration," making it an essential micronutrient for male fertility, according to the *Journal of Reproductive Infertility*.[5]

The research evidence for zinc supplementation, to support testosterone, provides mixed results. A study in the *Journal of Exercise Physiology* looked at the effects of a zinc/magnesium formulation on a group of test subjects, all competitive athletes, and identified a large increase in free testosterone, along with an increase in muscle strength.[6]

Another study, however, this one in the *European Journal of Clinical Nutrition*, used a group of healthy exercising men and investigated the impact of a zinc nutritional supplement on their serum testosterone levels and found "no significant effects regarding serum testosterone levels and the metabolism of testosterone in subjects who consume a zinc-sufficient diet." It's important to note that this study was with men who already had a normal zinc diet and zinc levels in their body, so future research might focus on men who are zinc and testosterone deficient.[7]

Is High Zinc Intake Related to Prostate Cancer?

Prostate cancer is the second leading cause of death among men in the United States, with more than one hundred eighty thousand new cases diagnosed each year. Some early studies of zinc intake and this type of cancer found indications of a causal association, but the results were inconsistent. So more research has been done.

In a 2009 study of 35,242 men published in the journal *Nutrition Cancer*, their ten-year average intake of zinc was measured against prostate cancer occurrence. The cancer researchers concluded that "long-term supplemental zinc intake was associated with reduced risk of clinically relevant advanced disease. . . . Risk of advanced prostate cancer decreased with greater intake of supplemental zinc."[8]

African American men have higher prostate cancer rates (a 60 percent higher risk) and a higher mortality than white men. To determine whether their zinc consumption might provide a clue as to why, a review of the science study literature was conducted in 2016. It evaluated the findings of studies among African American men, aged forty to eighty-five years, and the results determined "there is no evidence for an association between zinc intake and prostate cancer."[9]

Other research discovered that zinc levels in the prostate are 83 percent lower when cancer is present in the gland, and zinc is 63 percent lower in the prostate when BPH is present, compared to normal prostate tissues. More research needs to be done to determine why zinc declines in the presence of cancer or BPH before recommendations can be made, or conclusions drawn, that zinc supplementation might prevent these medical conditions.[10]

Natural Solution: Nettle Root
(*Urtica dioica*)

A science study on stinging nettle root and benign prostatic hyperplasia was done with 558 patients, who reported symptomatic benign prostatic hyperplasia. Their conditions were evaluated based on urinary flow, residual urine volume, serum prostatic-specific antigen (PSA), testosterone levels, and prostate size.

At the end of six months, patients who had received a placebo treatment were switched over to the stinging nettle root (*Urtica dioica*) supplement group and the study continued for another eighteen months. Eighty-one percent of those patients taking the supplement saw improved lower urinary tract symptoms, their overall prostate symptoms scores improved, urine flow rates improved, and there was no change in their serum PSA and testosterone levels.[11]

A lab animal study published in 2012 in the science journal *Andrologia* also found benefits from use of the herb, concluding that the study results "led us to conclude that *Urtica dioica* (stinging nettle) can be used as an effective drug for the management of BPH."[12]

Natural Solution: Saw Palmetto (*Serenoa repens*)

Results from scientific studies evaluating whether berry extracts of the American saw palmetto, or dwarf palm plant, can be effective in treating BPH, have been mixed and inconsistent, at best.

In the *Journal of Urology*, in 2000, scientists at the UCLA School of Medicine tested a saw palmetto herbal blend in forty-four men, forty-five to eighty years old. The science team reported the following from their findings: "Saw palmetto herbal blend appears to be a safe, highly desirable option for men with moderately symptomatic BPH. The secondary outcome measures of clinical effect in our study were only slightly better for saw palmetto herbal blend than placebo [not statistically significant]." However, in the aftermath of participating in this study, forty-one of the forty-four male participants "elected to continue therapy in an open label extension," basically endorsing their satisfaction with the treatment.[13]

Georgetown University Medical Center scientists tested a blend of natural products (saw palmetto, cernitin, B-sitosterol, and vitamin E) in treating symptoms of BPH in seventy patients in the intervention group and compared the results with fifty-seven patients in the placebo group. The clinical trial lasted three months. At the end of the study, those receiving the herbal blend reported a "highly significant" positive effect in BPH, based on the American Urological Association Symptom Index score.[14]

Contrast the previous studies with the results of a 2012 study review that evaluated the findings of several clinical trials of saw palmetto for treatment of BPH. The study review came to the conclusion that saw palmetto "at double and triple doses, did not improve urinary flow measures or prostate size in men with lower urinary tract symptoms consistent with BPH."[15]

Why is there such an inconsistency in these science results? Two studies from 2016 and 2017 offer a possible explanation.

In the 2016 study, Italian urologists did a series of tests on the effects of saw palmetto, along with selenium and lycopene (an antioxidant found in red and pink fruits), on symptoms of BPH. They didn't find evidence that saw palmetto was effective by itself: "the use of [saw palmetto] in BPH/LUTS (lower urinary tract symptoms) is not sustained by clear evidence for a therapeutic efficacy." But when saw palmetto was mixed with selenium and lycopene, a positive impact on symptoms was documented.[16]

The 2017 review of saw palmetto study results, published in the *Journal of Alternative and Complementary Medicine*, speculated that the herbal remedy benefitted from a "strong placebo effect, potentially influenced by positive patients' expectation on saw palmetto, shapes both the clinical practice outcomes and the findings of clinical trials." But beyond this imaginary positive psychological effect among users, when saw palmetto is combined with other herbal ingredients, there may be "potential synergistic effects." In other words, the various ingredients in the herbs interact with each other to produce therapeutic effects on BPH symptoms, making saw palmetto useful in these combinations, though not as a treatment on its own, except as a placebo.[17]

Natural Solution: Pumpkin Seed Oil Extract (*Cucurbita pepo*)

Pumpkin seed, which is rich in zinc, has a history of use as a natural alternative to pharmaceutical drugs, and its usefulness has been affirmed by scientific studies.

A major urology science journal published a study in 2015, out of Germany, involving 1,431 men, aged fifty to eighty years, diagnosed with BPH who were randomly assigned to one of two test groups:

pumpkin seed capsules with pumpkin seed extract or a placebo control group. After twelve months of study, the science team was able to determine that "treatment with pumpkin seed led to a clinically relevant reduction in IPSS (International Prostate Symptom Score) compared with placebo."[18]

Another urology science journal, in 2016, analyzed the results from sixteen studies that had tested the impact of pumpkin seed supplementation on patients with BPH. The study findings comparison showed that pumpkin seed had an anti-inflammatory effect producing "an improvement in International Prostatic Symptoms Score and a reduction in prostate growth."[19]

Natural Solution: Testosterone Replacement Therapy

Into the twenty-first century, many urologists and mainstream physicians warned their patients against undertaking testosterone replacement therapy because of an alleged risk of triggering or worsening BPH symptoms and, more seriously, also possibly causing prostate cancer. These cautions generated widespread anxiety and prevented untold thousands of men with low testosterone from taking advantage of the health benefits of replacement therapy. These concerns were thoroughly addressed and persuasive dispelled in a series of science studies over the last half-decade.

University of Washington Department of Medicine scientists did a study of male military veterans, aged forty to eighty-nine years, who had low testosterone and some of whom were treated with replacement therapy. The science team published their results in 2018, showing that among 147,593 men, "no association between cumulative testosterone dose or formulation and prostate cancer was observed."[20]

A similar finding came in a *British Journal of Urology* study, in 2017, in which thirty-six months of assessments were performed with 999 men with clinically diagnosed low testosterone, among whom 750 initiated replacement therapy. Over the study period, the percentage of men in each group—testosterone treated and untreated—developing prostate cancer was the same. There were also no differences in overall PSA levels or IPSS (International Prostate Symptom Score) in the two groups. "Results support prostate safety of TRT (testosterone replacement therapy) in newly diagnosed men with HG (low testosterone)," the journal reported.[21]

At the David Geffen School of Medicine at UCLA, scientists in the Department of Urology published findings, in a study review, that laid out how "a paradigm shift" had occurred in the field of urology as "recent data has changed the way we approach the treatment of testosterone deficiency in men with prostate cancer." According to these specialists, writing in a 2017 issue of *Current Urology Reports*, "The conventional notion that defined the relationship between increasing testosterone and prostate cancer growth was based on limited studies and anecdotal case reports. Contemporary evidence suggests testosterone therapy in men with testosterone deficiency does not increase prostate cancer risk or the chances of more aggressive disease at prostate cancer diagnosis. This led to a paradigm shift that testosterone therapy might in fact be a viable option for a select group of men with testosterone deficiency and a concurrent diagnosis of prostate cancer."[22]

As further evidence, another study review, also in *Current Urology Reports*, this time detailing myths about the relationship between BPH and testosterone, reported, "Contrary to the previous dogma that prostatic growth is directly proportional to testosterone levels, emerging research has suggested a lack of testosterone may be a risk factor of lower urinary tract symptoms (LUTS) and benign prostatic hyperplasia (BPH). The current evidence suggests that not only does testosterone replacement therapy (TRT) not worsen LUTS, but that hypogonadism [low testosterone] itself is an important risk factor for LUTS/BPH."[23]

Finally, we have this analysis from the Department of Urology at Tulane University: "TRT [testosterone replacement therapy] may improve components of the metabolic syndrome, which is associated with worsening LUTS [lower urinary tract symptoms]. Furthermore, the evidence suggests that TRT may decrease prostatic inflammation, which is also associated with worsening LUTS. The data on the relationship between TRT and LUTS have never shown worsening of LUTS, often shown no change in LUTS, and occasionally shown improvement."[24]

Since most studies have also found no prostate gland growth after long-term testosterone replacement, as a result, some men with enlarged prostates can qualify for testosterone therapy. Only a physician can make the final decision, and it's also advisable for a physician to monitor prostate health with regular PSA blood tests.

Restoring Male Sexual Function 15

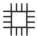

S EXUAL DYSFUNCTION OFTEN BECOMES the norm when a man is in the throes of andropause. Some of the most common symptoms of a man whose testosterone levels are declining are that he no longer wakes up in the morning with an erection, his erections take longer to achieve and are less firm, he may no longer feel sexual desire, and his penis and scrotum may even undergo shrinkage from testosterone deprivation.

A lot of scientific evidence supports the link between testosterone decline and erectile dysfunction. To illustrate, a 2015 study in the *Journal of Sexual Medicine* involving 733 men, aged twenty-one to forty years, found in this rather youthful age group that low testosterone clearly equaled erectile dysfunction. If the men had both low free testosterone and high sex hormone–binding globulin (SHBG), their risk for experiencing erectile dysfunction was even higher.[1]

Estradiol, the predominant form of estrogen in both female and male bodies, also plays an important role in male sexual function, affecting libido (sexual desire) as well as erections, according to urologists at the University of Miami, Department of Urology. Writing in a 2016 science journal study, they describe how "low testosterone and elevated estrogen increase the incidence of erectile dysfunction independently of one another."[2]

This strong connection between erectile dysfunction, sexual desire, and low testosterone was documented vividly in a study published in the *New England Journal of Medicine*. A research team provided 198 healthy men, twenty to fifty years of age, with a substance (goserelin acetate) to suppress testosterone and estradiol. Half the men were then assigned to receive a placebo gel, and the other half were administered a testosterone gel daily for sixteen weeks.

The scientists reported in their study, "Sexual desire decreased progressively with declining testosterone doses, from 10 g to 0 g of testosterone daily. Erectile function worsened significantly in men who received placebo, as compared with men who received testosterone, and declined more in men who received 1.25 g of testosterone daily than in men in the three highest dose groups."[3]

We detailed earlier in this book how a loss of sleep reduces testosterone levels in males and how both obesity and metabolic syndrome also have this same testosterone-lowering effect. Furthermore, study evidence indicates all of these conditions are causally linked to erectile dysfunction. "Sleep loss reduces testosterone levels in males and low sex steroid hormone concentrations have been associated with sexual dysfunction," reported a study in the science journal *Brain Research*.[4] "Metabolic Syndrome (MetS) has been associated with hypogonadism and erectile dysfunction (ED) and MetS may be considered a risk factor for ED," declared the *Journal of Andrology*.[5]

The biochemical pathways connecting testosterone deficiency to erectile dysfunction and impaired libido have yet to be clearly delineated. There are so many apparent direct and indirect interconnections between sexual dysfunction in men and the testosterone depletions caused by andropause, sleep disruption, chronic stress, metabolic syndrome, and obesity, all combined, that treatment by a holistic approach of solutions seems more than warranted. It seems mandatory.

Treatment of erectile dysfunction is also important for other reasons related to overall health and disease prevention. Every man should be made aware that there is a distinct connection between erectile dysfunction and the development of cardiovascular disease (CVD). A 2013 review of study findings determined that erectile dysfunction (ED) in men with no known CVD, often precedes the man having a cardiovascular event by two to five years, with the severity of the ED being correlated with increasing plaque burden. This is most true among men aged thirty to sixty years.[6]

RESTORING MALE SEXUAL FUNCTION 117

Since we can think of the penis as a type of hydraulic organ, sensitive to vascular blood flow disturbances, it makes sense that if you experience plaque build-up in your body's blood vessels, this plaque will affect the small vessels of the penis first, impairing their pliability.[7]

Shockwave Treatment for Erectile Dysfunction

Within the past decade or so a noninvasive technological advancement has emerged for the treatment of erectile dysfunction that promises benefits for men without causing any side effects. It involves a device that emits low-intensity shock waves to restore blood vessel function in the penis, revitalizing the erectile mechanism to better enable spontaneous erections to occur.

A review of the study evidence for this device, published in the science journal *Therapeutic Advances in Urology*, declared, "The results of our studies, which also included a double-blind randomized control trial, confirm that low-intensity extracorporeal shock wave therapy generates a significant clinical improvement of erectile function and a significant improvement in penile hemodynamics without any adverse effects."

The device "is a revolutionary treatment of ED," continued the study article, "and probably possesses unprecedented qualities that can rehabilitate erectile tissue. . . . It may create a new standard of care for men with ED."[8]

Natural Solution: Exercise Intervention

It is well documented that obesity and physical inactivity have a direct association with low testosterone and erectile dysfunction. Studies in the *Journal of Sexual Medicine* and the *British Journal of Sports Medicine* have explored these interconnections in a range of studies within the past decade.

Ninety abdominally obese men, with an age range of thirty to sixty years, were assigned to either a low volume or a high volume of moderate-intensity exercise to measure the effect on sexual function, testosterone levels, and lower urinary tract symptoms. The study lasted for twenty-four weeks. The study authors found that "moderate-intensity aerobic exercise of more than two hundred minutes [per] week produces greater improvements in sexual function, testosterone, weight, waist circumference and fat mass" than lower volumes of exercise or doing no exercise. These increases in all scoring parameters were labeled "significantly greater" in positive impact on all of the men involved.[9]

A group of scientists from Portugal undertook a systematic review of worldwide study results on exercise and erectile function in 2017. They uncovered "a statistically significant improvement in erectile function score" from aerobic exercise of a moderate-to-vigorous intensity. A benefit to sexual function was detected in both short-term and long-term exercise interventions.[10]

Natural Solution: The Mediterranean Diet

Previously, we noted that research has found the Mediterranean diet to be effective in treating obesity and metabolic disorder. Now we can add to that studies showing it improves erectile dysfunction (ED).

Let's start with two studies from 2010, both published in the *Journal of Sexual Medicine*. One study was done among men thirty-five to seventy years of age, with a diagnosis of type 2 diabetes and erectile dysfunction. A total of 555 men were involved. It was determined that those men with the greatest adherence to the Mediterranean diet had a lower prevalence of ED.[11]

The second study was a systematic scientific literature review on the subject of diet and ED among men. Findings from the various studies were in agreement that the "Mediterranean diet was more effective than a control diet in ameliorating ED or restoring absent ED in people with obesity or metabolic disorder."[12]

Italian scientists writing in the science journal *Urologia* revealed in 2017 how they examined 141 patients with ED and divided them into two study groups: one on the Mediterranean diet, the other not on it. Using the International Index of Erectile Function, they monitored and measured both groups before, during, and after the study period. The science team concluded, "Adherence to Med-Diet showed a significant difference between the two groups" affording adherents "protective factors against ED."[13]

Finally, in a Canadian study of fruit and vegetable consumption and erectile dysfunction among men with diabetes, scientists reported that "a 10% risk reduction of ED was found with each additional serving of fruit/vegetable consumed." This protective effect against ED was reinforced the more these men stuck to a vegetarian or vegan diet.[14]

It should also be noted that traditional Chinese medicine and the Ayurvedic tradition of India have long considered ginger, garlic, and fava beans helpful in treating erectile dysfunction, because all three are known to promote blood flow in the lower body.

Among natural plant-based testosterone enhancers, we have celery, which has historically been seen as a medicinal plant whose chemical makeup gives it a wide range of health-affirming effects: antimicrobial, antibacterial, and anti-inflammatory. It's been used as a remedy for urinary problems, gout, arthritis, high blood pressure, and also as a sexual tonic for men and their reproductive system.

Natural Solution: Vitamin D Supplementation

A body of science data emerged in 2017 and 2018 demonstrating a link between low vitamin D and low testosterone and how supplementation with vitamin D can be beneficial to male sexual health.

The first study appeared in the science journal *Aging Male*. A group of 102 male patients, average age of fifty-three years, were included in the twelve-month-long experiment using vitamin D supplements. The science team reported, "This study demonstrated that VD (vitamin D) treatment improves testosterone levels, metabolic syndrome and erectile function in middle-aged men."[15]

A second study in 2018, this one published in the *International Journal of Endocrinology*, studied 114 men for a possible association between vitamin D and sexual function. "After vitamin D replacement therapy," the scientists observed, "total and free testosterone increased and erectile function improved." The higher the levels of vitamin D administered, the better the observed improvements in erectile function.[16]

However, these results need to be contrasted with a third study, published in the *European Journal of Nutrition*, that also measured the impact of vitamin D supplementation on testosterone levels. In this research, 100 men were randomized into a control placebo group and an intervention vitamin D group for twelve weeks. "We found no significant treatment effect on serum total testosterone," the Austrian scientists wrote.[17] Why the testosterone results from these various vitamin D studies were in conflict needs to be resolved by future research examining possible confounding factors.

Natural Solution: Maca Root (*Lepidium meyenii*)

For centuries in the Andean cultures of Peru, and for decades in Western herbal medicine, maca root, found high in the central Andes, has been extolled for its alleged aphrodisiac and fertility-enhancing effects in men and women. While maca root science testing in women has shown some beneficial effects, the record of findings is more checkered among men.

In a twelve-week clinical trial among men between twenty-one and fifty-six years of age, published in the *Journal of Endocrinology*, maca supplementation was tested for its effects on male hormones. The result: "Data showed that compared with placebo, Maca had no effect on any of the hormones studied nor did the hormones show any changes over time. Treatment with Maca does not affect serum reproductive hormone levels."[18]

In a 2018 study published in the *Journal of Ethnopharmacology*, British scientists did a study review of research on maca root to evaluate findings related to its effects on male sexual health. Their conclusion: "So far, the in vivo studies and clinical trials conducted have yielded inconclusive results. . . . The health claims of maca cannot be fully supported from a scientific standpoint."[19]

Natural Solution: Puncture Vine (*Tribulus terrestris*)

From the Ayurveda medicine tradition springs this hairy leaf plant with yellow flowers whose leaf extracts have been considered an aphrodisiac for centuries by herbalists from India and China. Scientific evidence has thus far found it to be more effective in women than men in simulating libido and sexual function, but the results in men, especially in awakening the libido and boosting erections, were beneficial enough to warrant inclusion here.

An extensive review of the scientific literature on this plant was carried out in the *Journal of Ethnopharmacology* in 2016, and the studies done in both humans and animals revealed "an important role for *Tribulus terrestris* in treating erectile dysfunction and sexual desire problems."[20]

A second study review of evidence for the plant's beneficial effects on sexual function, conducted by Chinese scientists in 2017, explained why this plant "over the last several years, has been certified for its pharmaceutical activities [in China] for improving sexual function." The variety of saponins and flavonoids, bioactive phytochemicals, identified in the plant were analyzed for their various pharmacological activities in the human body.[21] At first, scientists thought the plant acted on the human body by mimicking or influencing the sex hormones of both men and women. Later research has centered on a mechanism by which the plant synthesizes nitric oxide, another compound affecting sexual function.

Natural Solution: Thai Black Ginger (*Kaempferia parviflora*)

Another ancient traditional herbal aphrodisiac, this medicinal plant is found in northeastern parts of Thailand. It's also called Thai ginseng. A 2017 study using healthy elderly male volunteers found 61.5 percent of them had improvement in their erections from using this plant extract. "The treatment demonstrated improvement in certain study parameters related to erectile function and male sexual health," the study authors concluded.[22]

During a test of KaempMax, an ethanol extract of the plant, scientists writing in the *Journal of Integrative Medicine* in 2018 described how its use over thirty days in males aged fifty to sixty-eight years "resulted in statistically significant improvements in erectile function, intercourse satisfaction, and total scores" on a sexual function scale (International Index of Erectile Function). It was well tolerated by the volunteers, showed no side effects, and seemed to exercise its effects in both the brain and the body.[23]

Natural Solution: Malaysian Ginseng (*Eurycoma longifolia*)

Roots of this flowering plant have long been touted historically as having aphrodisiac, erectile function, and testosterone-enhancing effects, some of which have been subsequently affirmed in science lab testing.

In the science journal *Andrologia*, a study appeared in which seventy-six men with late-onset hypogonadism (low testosterone) were given 200 mg a day of a water-soluble extract of the herb for one month. Serum testosterone levels were measured before, during, and after, as were the aging males symptoms for andropause.

The study team concluded, "Results show that treatment significantly improved the Ageing Males Symptoms score (71.7% had normal values after treatment) as well as the serum testosterone concentration (90.8% of the patients showed normal values after treatment)."[24]

In 2014, *Andrologia* again reported, "Eurycoma longifolia is a natural alternative to testosterone replacement therapy and has been shown to restore serum testosterone levels, thus significantly improving sexual health. This includes significant positive effects on bone health and physical condition of patients. Thus far, at therapeutic concentrations, no significant side effects of the treatment were obvious. Therefore, it might be a safe alternative to testosterone treatment therapy."[25]

A review of the clinical trial study literature for this herb in the journal *Complementary Therapeutic Medicine* uncovered evidence of "significant improvement" in erectile function in those test subjects who began with the lowest baseline erectile functions scores when the studies began.[26]

Natural Solution: Korean Red Ginseng

Long known for its effectiveness in treating sexual function in menopausal women, this herb has also received scientific attention for its effects on erectile dysfunction and overall sexual satisfaction in men. One of the first Korean red ginseng and ED studies in a reputable science journal, the *Journal of Urology*, appeared back in 2002, in which forty-five patients with clinically diagnosed erectile dysfunction were enrolled in an eighteen-week clinical trial. Those in the intervention group received 900 mg of Korean red ginseng, three times a day; those in the control group received a placebo.

At the conclusion of the study, 60 percent of patients in the ginseng intervention group reported improved erections. Penile rigidity also showed "significant improvement" compared to the placebo group. "Our data show that Korean red ginseng can be an effective alternative [to pharmaceutical drugs] for treating male erectile dysfunction," the science team declared.[27]

Sixty patients with mild to moderate ED were enrolled in a 2007 clinical trial study, comparing Korean red ginseng to a placebo. The ginseng group received 1,000 mg three times a day. After twelve weeks, the ginseng group had "significantly higher" scores than the placebo group on the International Index of Erectile Function. The researchers wrote in the *Asian Journal of Andrology*, "Our data show that Korean Red Ginseng can be an effective alternative to the invasive approaches for treating male ED (erectile dysfunction)."[28]

The *British Journal of Clinical Pharmacology* published study review results in 2008 showing that among seven randomized clinical trials, the collective findings provided "suggestive evidence for the effectiveness of red ginseng in the treatment of erectile dysfunction."[29]

Finally, the *International Journal of Impotence Research* published results of a study of 119 men with mild to moderate ED. Participants were divided into two groups and administered either four tablets a day of Korean ginseng berry extract (350 mg per tablet) or a placebo, daily for eight weeks. The science team concluded that not only was the extract safe, but it also "improved all domains of sexual function. It can be used as an alternative medicine to improve sexual life in men with sexual dysfunction."[30]

As discussed in this chapter, there are a few herbs shown to support hormone balance and sexual performance in men. Quite possibly, using a combination of a few of these could reap synergistic benefits beyond using them alone. Four great options would be Korean red ginseng, puncture vine, maca, and horny goat weed. The latter is an ancient Chinese remedy containing icariin, a bioactive compound, which has been studied for its anti-inflammatory and erectile function support.

Natural Solution: Fenugreek
(*Trigonella foenum-graecum*)

Different formulation extracts, both derived from the fiber-rich fenugreek plant, have been developed in laboratories for use in treating sexual function in males. The first is called Testofen; the second is Furosap.

Sixty healthy males, age range twenty-five to fifty-two years, participated in a study testing whether Testofen, a standardized fenugreek extract and mineral formulation, could improve sexual function. They were given two tablets per day, 600 mg per tablet, for six weeks. The verdict at study's end: "It was concluded that Testofen demonstrated a significant positive effect on physiological aspects of libido and may assist to maintain normal healthy testosterone levels."[31]

A second study of Testofen, done in 2016 and published in the journal *Aging Male*, was a double-blind, randomized, placebo-controlled trial involving 120 healthy men, aged forty-three to seventy years of age. The intervention group received a dose of 600 mg of the extract a day, for twelve weeks. As the scientists reported, "Sexual function improved [in the intervention group] including number of morning erections and frequency of sexual activity. Both total serum testosterone and free testosterone increased compared to placebo after twelve weeks of active treatment. Trigonella foenum-graecum seed extract is a safe and effective treatment for reducing symptoms of possible androgen deficiency, improves sexual function and increases serum testosterone in healthy middle-aged and older men."[32]

The second treatment using an extract of fenugreek is a more recent laboratory innovation. In 2017, a research team based at universities in both the United States and India reported results of a clinical trial involving fifty men, aged thirty-five to sixty-five years old. They received 500 mg a day of Furosap over a twelve-week period. Results reported were as follows: "Free testosterone levels were improved up to 46% in [nine-tenths] of the study population," and the libidos improved in the majority of study subjects. No side effects of treatment were observed.[33]

Natural Solution: Ojayeonjonghwan

With major ingredients taken from five plants, including *Cornus officinalis* (a species of dogwood), the Korean herbal formulation called ojayeonjonghwan has been studied extensively, though for less than a decade, for its improvement of erectile dysfunction and other low-testosterone symptoms.

In a 2017 series of test tube and animal experiments, scientists writing in the science journal *Oxidative Medicine and Cellular Longevity* described how their results show the formulation offers "credible evidence for the use of new alternative therapies to treat late onset-hypogonadism symptoms, such as erectile dysfunction."[34]

A year later, scientists tested the herbal formulation in seventy-eight men who were randomly assigned to either an herbal intervention group or a control group with no treatment. After eight weeks, it was found that the treatment group significantly improved their sexual function and satisfaction scores. According to the resulting study report in the journal *Aging Male*, the herbal formulation "was found to be effective in all late-onset hypogonadism symptoms" and "may be safely used for treatment."[35]

In 2019, more animal testing confirmed the earlier findings that the herbal formulation "might be an effective alternative for [treating] late onset hypogoandism" because it increases the levels of serum testosterone and acts as an antioxidant to support testicular tissue.[36]

Natural Solution: VigRX Plus Supplement

This multiherbal oral supplement for the treatment of erectile dysfunction is a proprietary formula that mixes eight herbs: *Panax ginseng, Serenoa repens, Gingko biloba, Crateagus laevigate, Ptychopetalum olacoides, Erythroxylum catuaba, Cuscuta chinensis,* and *Epimedium sagittatum* extract. In a 2012 study, its safety and effectiveness was examined in seventy-eight men, aged twenty-five to fifty years of age, who reported mild to moderate severity in erectile dysfunction. They were divided into two groups: the first took two capsules daily of VigRX Plus for twelve weeks, and the second group received a placebo.

At the conclusion of the study, six scientists coauthored a report in the science journal *BMC Complementary Alternative Medicine* noting how test subjects using the supplement "improved significantly" their erectile function, as well as their orgasmic function, sexual desire, and overall satisfaction, compared to the placebo group.

On top of that, at study's end 90 percent of the supplement group elected to continue with the supplement treatment they had received. No side effects were reported.[37]

Natural Solution: Testosterone Replacement Therapy

Scientists in the Department of Urology at Baylor College of Medicine in Houston decided to test the impact of testosterone replacement on sexual function, using 271 patients with low testosterone and unsatisfactory sexual function. The experiment lasted twelve months and involved daily applications of Testim, a testosterone 1 percent topical gel.

At the end of the study period, a patient evaluation found that both total testosterone and free testosterone levels had improved significantly and all domains of measurement—sex drive/libido, erectile function, ejaculatory function—had also improved significantly, giving the research team the evidence it needed to recommend this replacement therapy.[38]

German scientists did a similar study in 2014, testing 261 men diagnosed with late-onset hypogonadism and erectile dysfunction. They were given testosterone undecanoate intramuscular injections of 1,000 mg a day. The study lasted five years. "Testosterone undecanoate treatment resulted in a sustained improvement in erectile function and muscle and joint pain, which contributed to an improvement in long-term health-related quality of life," the researchers concluded when publishing their results in the *Journal of Sexual Medicine*. Improvements were also noted in body weight, waist circumference, body mass index, lowered total cholesterol, and lowered blood pressure.[39]

A huge team of more than two dozen scientists, participating in a series of studies known as the Testosterone Trials, reported on their results in a 2015 science article published in the *Journal of Clinical Endocrinology & Metabolism*. Based on having worked with 788 study participants, sixty-five years of age and older, the research team saw supplementation raised free testosterone and total testosterone levels and that, in turn, "consistently, independently, and positively" raised measures of sexual desire, erectile function, and sexual activity.[40]

Even more of these Testosterone Trial results (there were seven trials in all) were released in 2016 in the same science journal, this time involving another group of 470 men, sixty-five years of age and older, who had been assigned to a testosterone (intervention) gel group or a placebo group for one year. At study's end, the intervention group showed significant improvement in ten of twelve measures of sexual activity and performance.[41]

In the science journal *European Urology*, European scientists did their own review of fourteen studies on testosterone and sexual function, involving more than twenty-two hundred men, with an average age of sixty years. In 2017, they reported their analysis of consensus findings from the studies: "These results argue that sexual dysfunction should be considered a hallmark manifestation of T (testosterone) deficiency, since those symptoms can be significantly improved with normalization of serum T. We found that testosterone treatment significantly improves erectile dysfunction, as well as other aspects of sexual function, in men with testosterone deficiency."[42]

About Testosterone Replacement Therapy   **16**

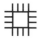

THROUGHOUT THIS BOOK we've presented references to testosterone replacement therapy (TRT) and examples of where the scientific evidence shows it to be effective in treating the symptoms of andropause. Whether the issue is weight loss, prostate health, or sexual dysfunction, we've first detailed and discussed an array of practical, effective, and safe natural treatments for these symptoms before leading you to TRT as a proven option.

Being nutritional practitioners, as a general rule we recommend trying and exhausting all natural treatment options before embracing any invasive treatment promoted by traditional medicine. Although TRT can be invasive if you choose an injectable form, it otherwise represents a safer and more effective alternative to the surgery or pharmaceutical drugs promoted by mainstream medicine for treating most andropause symptoms.

A testosterone-boosting natural treatment plan of your own creation might include such combined elements as resistance training, dietary intervention for weight loss and weight maintenance, and targeted supplementation. Each of these elements on their own can raise testosterone levels. To cite just a few examples:

- Use a "green drink" daily in combination with a high-energy (vegan) dietary program. A twenty-one-day study examined this approach with a group of men and women, in which they ate vegan meals three times a day along with a daily green drink composed of alfalfa, wheatgrass, and apple cider vinegar. Results showed a large increase in testosterone for the men, along with weight loss and improvements in cholesterol.[1]

- Or consider this supplementation example using garlic. An experiment with lab animals published in the *Journal of Nutrition* found strong evidence that daily dietary supplementation with a garlic powder greatly increased testicular testosterone. These results prompted the Japanese science team to recommend garlic supplements to men with low testosterone.[2]

- Velvet bean (*Mucuna pruriens*) grows on trees and has been used as an herbal remedy for fertility for generations in Ayurvedic medicine. Scientists in 2009 tested it in seventy-five fertile men and seventy-five men undergoing infertility screening. This herb was found to "significantly improve" testosterone and other hormone levels in infertile men, as well as sperm count.[3]

- Shilajit is another old Ayurvedic remedy, a tar-like resin found in rocks high in the Himalayan Mountains and containing up to eighty-five minerals. In the science journal *Andrologia*, a team of scientists tested it in men between forty-five and fifty-five years of age, administering a dose of 250 mg twice a day. After ninety days of treatment, it had "significantly increased total testosterone and free testosterone" in the test subjects.[4]

By combining and experimenting with these and other natural approaches, as outlined in this book, an entire lifestyle can be created with synergistic potential for the long-term increase and maintenance of optimal testosterone levels in the average male. As an adjunct to this approach, HRT can still play a supporting role to further enhance treatment effects for the entire range of andropause symptoms.

When all other natural solutions fail, there is a ready recourse of treatment involving hormone replacement. For men undergoing testosterone replacement therapy, positive effects are usually seen in three to six weeks. These benefits include improvements in attitude and sense of well-being; increased mental and physical energy; decreases in anger, irritability, sadness, and tiredness; improved sleep quality; improved libido and sexual performance; decline in biochemical markers of bone degradation; increases in lean body mass and a decline in fat; increased muscle strength; and a decreased heart disease risk.

Let's take a deeper dive into the subject of TRT and look at what TRT medications are available, their contrasting costs and safety profiles, and the many myths and concerns that have been expressed about this potent form of natural medicine.

Testosterone Replacement Therapy Options

If blood tests find that you are a candidate for hormone replacement therapy to "normalize" your levels, testosterone can be delivered into your body using a variety of mechanisms, the most common being skin patches, which allow a slow release of testosterone and are normally affixed to the abdomen, back, thighs, or upper arms; gels applied on or under the arms; capsules taken twice daily after meals; or injections of testosterone every two to four weeks.

"Proper use of bio-identical hormones must be individualized based on a patient's unique situation," cautions Florida urologist and hormone expert Dr. Kenneth Janson in an interview with our research associate, Randall Fitzgerald. "They should not be used until one has been carefully evaluated, and found to have suboptimal levels and a clinical indication for therapy. If therapy has been initiated, careful long-term monitoring of a patient's condition is critical, together with appropriate laboratory follow-up."

There is a myth that advancing age may preclude testosterone therapy, but that idea is disputed by some hormone specialists who say that no patient is too old to start testosterone therapy if it is clearly indicated by testing. It should be taken under a physician's care, with regular appropriate follow-up evaluations. A physician should also monitor the health of your prostate with regular PSA blood tests and physical examinations.

After three to six weeks of testosterone replacement therapy, some benefits that are often reported include increased mental and physical energy, less irritability, improved sleep quality, and greater libido. For men undergoing testosterone replacement therapy, positive effects are usually seen in three to six weeks.

One persistent myth about testosterone replacement is that it will "bring out the beast in men." This myth came about because of an overuse of high-dose testosterone replacement by certain men, mostly those with athletic or body-building aspirations, men who usually had normal testosterone levels to begin with but wanted to further enhance their self-image. This abuse of testosterone by young athletes has been widely publicized. It is usually done without proper medical guidance. Young athletes who have naturally high levels of testosterone and resort to using testosterone products are taking serious health risks, including infertility, testicular atrophy, emotional instability, and cardiovascular complications.

But for nonathletes with suboptimal testosterone levels, a wealth of data in authoritative medical journals shows strong evidence that low testosterone levels are associated with a *higher* risk of cardiovascular disease, diabetes, depression, sexual dysfunction, and cognitive decline.

Dr. Kenneth Janson, who prescribes testosterone to patients with suboptimal levels who medically qualify, cautions us not to confuse "normal" and "suboptimal." (Normal is often considered a range of 200ng/dL to 1100ng/dL.) He notes that when we get older, testosterone frequently becomes suboptimal, but it is still considered "normal." He says aging men often suffer the dual effects of too little testosterone and too much estrogen. The resulting imbalance causes many of the health problems associated with normal aging because as men age, testosterone increasingly converts to estrogen.

The option of undertaking reasonable testosterone therapy has sometimes been intentionally withheld from men who would benefit from this replacement therapy simply because the men didn't satisfy the accepted mainstream definition of what constitutes "low" levels of the hormone. Physicians who work daily with patients with low levels of testosterone know that statistical definitions of what is high and low are at the extremes and therefore a poor basis for deciding who is a candidate for therapy. The goal should be to return a man to his own "optimal" hormone levels of healthy, youthful physiology based on his individualized physiological needs.

Dr. Janson continues: "The key to using testosterone safely is to use it for appropriate indications in men who have been shown to have suboptimal levels, and make sure therapy is carefully monitored on an ongoing basis by a physician who has appropriate training in its proper use. A thorough medical history and careful physical examination should be prerequisites to any consideration of hormone therapy. Then after commencing therapy, a patient should have regular consultations with a physician, who should always give advice on proper nutrition, exercise, and lifestyle choices; monitor appropriate laboratory studies and overall clinical progress; and perform regular physical examinations."

A note of caution about hormone mills: Many "hormone mills" are operated by charlatans. They don't care about giving you dietary, exercise, and supplement education and support to strengthen your health and well-being. They only care about selling you a steady supply of testosterone.[5, 6, 7, 8]

Contrasting the TRT Delivery Systems

We've drawn from two primary authoritative sources for the TRT information detailed below: a 2017 comparison of TRT medications appearing in the *Journal for Nurse Practitioners*, prepared by professors at Brigham Young University, and a 2016 comparison of TRT formulations appearing in the science journal *Translational Andrology and Urology*.[9, 10]

Six types of delivery for TRT have been approved by the U.S. Food and Drug Administration: buccal (gum) absorption, intramuscular (injectable), nasal spray, subdermal pellets, transdermal gels/liquids, and transdermal patches. A seventh mode of delivery—formulations taken *orally*—has not been approved in the United States, due to its suspected toxic effects on the liver, but it is available elsewhere in the world.

Here is a background overview of all six delivery systems used, as of this writing, in the United States. Pricing is based on 2017 cost guides:

- **Buccal (Gum) Absorption**—An application of adhesive tablets to the gums of the mouth for absorption, this method received FDA approval in 2003 and has been marketed under

the brand name of Striant by Actient Pharmaceuticals. This
form of delivery bypasses the liver. One 30 mg dose tablet is
placed in the side of the mouth onto the gums every twelve
hours. Sixty tablets (each tablet 30 mg) were sold for an
average of $724.77 in 2017.

- **Intramuscular (Injectable)**—Since the 1950s, injectable
forms of testosterone have been on the market for direct
application to muscles. Three types of injection preparations
are FDA approved: testosterone cypionate (TC), testosterone
enanthate (TE), and testosterone undecanoate (TU). They
differ in their carbon chain chemical makeup. TC includes
Depo-Testosterone by Pfizer Inc., which may be the most
popular prescribed replacement therapy in the United States.
TE was first marketed in 1954, under the name of Delatestryl
by Endo Pharmaceuticals, as well as under many other brand
names. TU is branded as Aveed by Endo Pharmaceuticals
and also marketed under several other names. According to
2017 pricing, the average cost per month for the 100 mg/mL
Depo-Testosterone was $22.70; the 200 mg/mL was $98.07
a month. Delatestryl as a generic was available at 200 mg/mL
for $23.46 per month, on average.

- **Nasal Spray**—A nasal gel with applicator pump, approved
in 2014 by the FDA, is marketed under the name of Natesto
by Endo Pharmaceuticals. A pump delivers 5.5 mg of
testosterone, with a recommended application of three times
a day in the nostrils, giving a daily dose of 33 mg. Three
bottles, enough to last thirty days, went for an average of
$699.21 in 2017.

- **Subdermal Pellets**—These were introduced in the 1940s
and have been described as the first effective formulation for
testosterone replacement therapy. The pellets, in a 150–450
mg dose, are implanted in the hip or other fatty area at
three- to six-month intervals. Testopel marketed by Auxilium
Pharmaceuticals is a popular brand. Average cost per month of
pellets in 2017 was around $225, based on twelve to sixteen
pellets being implanted twice a year.

- **Transdermal Gels/Liquids**—Starting in 2002, gel and
liquid testosterone formulations received FDA approval, but

with a warning label (a U.S. "black box warning") due to the risk of skin contact of the wearer with others, particularly women and children. Popular gel brands include AndroGel by AbbVie Inc., Fortesta by Endo Pharmaceuticals, Testim by Auxilium Pharmaceuticals, and Vogelxo by Upsher-Smith Laboratories. A liquid solution in a metered-dose pump called Axiron is manufactured by Eli Lilly. AndroGel averaged $516.41 for a month's supply in 2017, compared to an average of $630.78 a month for Axiron.

- **Transdermal Patches**—First introduced in the 1980s, as scrotal patches, they have since been replaced in popularity, as a delivery mechanism, by patches applied to the thighs, upper arms, or abdomen. Non-scrotal patches include Androderm by Actavis, approved by the FDA in 1995. Starting doses are a single 4 mg patch applied every twenty-four hours. Thirty patches of Androderm went for an average of $195.03 in 2017.

Which of the TRT Methods Are Safest and Most Effective?

"When considering all available routes of delivery, concentrations, and branded or generic choices, there are currently over thirty different testosterone preparations to consider when choosing one for a patient," advised the 2016 *Translational Andrology and Urology* study article on TRT, referenced earlier. "The decision on the best product choice should include patient preferences, pharmacokinetics, treatment burden, cost and insurance coverage. Products may also need to be switched throughout TRT based upon patient response, preference and adverse effects."

Side effects, costs, and effectiveness in raising testosterone levels were evaluated and compared for the various TRT medication products by Brigham Young University scientists, based on results from science studies they accessed.

Some of the more pronounced side effects they identified and highlighted include the following:

- More than 32 percent of Striant patients (buccal absorption) reported gingivitis as a side effect.

- Androderm had the highest occurrence of side effects among the transdermals, with more than 50 percent of users reporting skin irritations.
- Depo-Testosterone is the longest-used of the TRTs, and this injectable has few side effects on record in connection with that use.

A number of other studies have produced important findings.

In a 2018 examination of the transdermal Androgel, based on the treatment of 401 men with topical applications for three months, the science journal *Urologia* reported, "Androgel is highly effective and safe in the management of androgen deficiency. Its use in patients with chronic prostatitis and hypogonadism results in an improvement in low urinary tract symptoms [and] symptoms of chronic prostatitis . . . and thus leads to significant improvements in the quality of life."[11]

A study review of Testim gel, published in the journal *Expert Opinions Pharmacotherapy*, found that "the most common adverse events associated with Testim gel were application-site reactions and moderately increased prostate-specific antigen levels. . . . Overall, the clinical evidence so far indicates that Testim gel is a safe and effective treatment option for daily use in the management of male hypogonadism."[12]

The safety and effectiveness of a new topical 2 percent gel therapy called Tgel was assessed in a 2018 issue of the science journal *Andrologia* in 127 men who were administered it over nine months. Results were as follows: "Significant improvements in sexual function and quality of life were noted. Subjects experienced few skin reactions without notable increases in prostate-specific antigen. [It] was efficacious with an acceptable safety profile."[13]

Finally, in a 2015 review of TRT methods, British scientists writing in the journal *Aging Male* evaluated the following: pellet implants, oral testosterone undecanoate (Testocaps), mesterolone (Proviron), testosterone gel (Testogel), testosterone scrotal cream (Andromen), and scrotal gel (Tostran). As a general verdict, the research team observed, "the testosterone preparations appear equally safe over prolonged periods, with either no change or improvement of cardiovascular risk factors, especially in lowering cholesterol and diastolic blood pressure. It is suggested that because of excessive reliance on laboratory measures of androgens and undue safety concerns, many men who could benefit from symptom relief . . . remain untreated."[14]

In their review of TRT pricing, the Brigham Young University team found the most cost-efficient TRTs were the injectable formulations of Depo-Testosterone and Delatestryl.

Based on study findings of effectiveness, the same science team recommended Depo-Testosterone as "a good first-line therapy option." A good second-line option recommended was Androderm patches, which have one of the highest ratings for effectiveness. If these two options aren't tolerated well by the patient, a third option recommended is Testim, the transdermal gel, which is both affordable and associated with some of the fewest reported side effects, so long as the user covers the treated area with clothing to avoid contaminating others.

Is Bioidentical TRT Superior to Synthetic TRT?

This is an ongoing debate in search of still more research evidence, which is an important process given that hormones are the messengers telling all the various parts of the human body what to do and when to do it. Having hormones out of balance can cause mixed or misinterpreted messages being sent throughout the body, triggering a range of serious symptoms of dysfunction.

The standard and best way to describe bioidentical hormones, whether they are testosterone used in men or estrogen and progesterone in women, is that they are derived from chemical precursors drawn primarily from plant sources, such as yam or soybean molecules, to be made as identical as possible to the hormones produced by the human body. These bioidentical products are commercially processed, but not synthesized using chemicals in a laboratory. As a result, bioidentical hormones can be customized to better fit a patient's body chemistry needs. These mixtures are generally made in what is known as compounding pharmacies.

By contrast, pharmaceutical-lab-synthesized replacement hormones emerge as standardized, whether for use in men or women.

Though some natural hormones derived from plant or animal sources may be used in some synthetic products, for the most part, these are lab-created chemical mixtures designed to resemble human hormones. Pharmaceutical scientists say they also modify testosterone's molecular structure in the lab to improve its bioavailability (its absorption rate into your body).

Nearly all of the scientific research done on bioidentical versus synthetic hormone replacement therapy benefits has been done by examining estrogen and progesterone. Little research has emerged directly comparing bioidentical to synthetic in the production, administration, safety, and effectiveness profiles of testosterone.

"Customized bioidentical hormones are often advertised as being a safer, more effective, natural, and an individualized alternative to conventional hormone therapy," reports the Cleveland Clinic, a nonprofit academic medical center. "However, these claims remain unsupported by any large-scale, well designed studies."[15]

Based on the limited research that has been undertaken, there is evidence that bioidentical hormones are a preferred treatment approach. Though this research comparing bioidentical to synthetic was done with three hormones generally given to women, we suspect it also has comparable applications to the differences in testosterone replacement seen in bioidentical versus synthetic.

A study review published in the journal *Postgraduate Medicine* evaluated the research done comparing the effects of bioidentical and synthetics (estradiol, estriol, and progesterone) and their levels of safety and patient satisfaction. "Bioidentical hormones have some distinctly different, potentially opposite, physiological effects compared with their synthetic counterparts, which have different chemical structures," observed the study review. "Physiological data and clinical outcomes demonstrate that bioidentical hormones are associated with lower risks . . . and are more efficacious than their synthetic and animal-derived counterparts. Until evidence is found to the contrary, bioidentical hormones remain the preferred method of HRT [hormone replacement therapy]. Further randomized controlled trials are needed to delineate these differences more clearly."[16]

While it may be true that more studies and deeper research needs to be done, in the meantime, while consumers are waiting for conclusive results, they must choose whether to use bioidentical hormones or synthetic ones. Our observation and experience with the bioidentical option convinces us to recommend it as a preferred hormone replacement delivery choice.

Is Blood Testing the Most Viable Way to Measure Hormone Levels?

To customize bioidentical hormones, saliva testing is used rather than a reliance on blood testing, to determine hormone levels and individual needs. Some mainstream medical institutions object to that approach.

The Mayo Clinic, on its website, for instance, writes that bioidentical hormones are "custom-made for you, based on a test of your saliva to assess your unique hormonal needs. Unfortunately, however, the hormone levels in your saliva don't reflect the levels in your blood."[17]

We beg to differ with that assessment, if only based on the experience of one of our colleagues: Dr. Paul Ling Tai, who is a recognized expert in this hormone testing realm. Dr. Tai is the chairman of the Department of Post Graduate Medical Education and chairman of the Department of Medical Research at University of Health Science Antigua, School of Medicine and School of Nursing. He has also been head research coordinator of a multicenter clinical correlation study on endocrinology and saliva test, a co-project with the University of UniAmericas, Brazil. By collecting multiple saliva samples during the day, a much more accurate hormone level reading can be taken and measured than by using blood samples or a single saliva test.

"As a physician with special attention to anti-aging medicine, my therapeutic preference starts with a saliva hormone test to establish a baseline for all natural supplemental treatment," wrote Dr. Tai in the magazine published by our own Hippocrates Health Institute. He is on our advisory board and consults with our medical team.[18]

> Why go through the trouble of an invasive blood test when you can effortlessly collect five saliva samples and receive quicker, more accurate results? The idea that blood testing is the be-all-end-all to determining the levels in our bodies is a misconception. In fact, saliva is directly produced from blood, but has been filtered of any bound hormones that can interfere with accurate test results.

Blood or serum level measurements are numbers that are affected by bound hormones, even though your body will never actually absorb them. The "free" hormones, also called bio-available hormones, are the ones that are available to affect your body, your energy levels, your libido and your life. By exclusively testing free hormones, you are given a more accurate point of reference for your health and treatment.

These free hormones are able to easily cross the salivary gland wall, where the bound hormones are too heavy to breach the membrane barriers due to their molecular weight. Saliva is perfect to test for hormones due to active and free hormones being constantly present in samples. Accurately measuring free hormone levels is essential to diagnosing, planning, and maintaining proper treatment, as well as balancing hormones for total health.

Will TRT Stimulate Prostate Growth and Cancer?

Whether testosterone replacement therapy can trigger prostate growth and subsequently prostate cancer was a longtime point of contention between scientists, in the field of urology in particular as well as mainstream medicine in general.

What initiated these concerns and the debate was a medical finding, in 1941, that male castration leads to prostate cancer regression because testosterone is no longer present. That set in motion the idea of high testosterone levels being linked to the onset of prostate cancer.[19]

Throughout the remainder of the twentieth century, as testosterone replacement therapy emerged as a method of treating the low testosterone levels in andropausal men, studies on this suspected link between prostate cancer and testosterone showed decidedly mixed results. Some studies showed no linkage; others produced results indicating a connection existed. Confusion reigned, and so caution prevailed, with the U.S. Food and Drug Administration mandating that warning labels be affixed on all testosterone products.

A key reason why negative study findings had emerged showing a linkage was identified by the *Journal of Urology* in 2015. "Much of this controversy appears to be based on conflicting study designs, definitions, and methodologies. Contradictory findings have been reported largely due to the disparate methodologies used in many studies. Most studies [finding a testosterone/cancer link] did not adhere to professional society guidelines on total testosterone measurements."[20]

Once the study methodologies were brought more into alignment, research findings on testosterone and the prostate became more consistent, showing there to be little cancer risk for men in undergoing testosterone replacement therapy.

For example, the science journal *European Urology* published a study review of testosterone replacement therapy in which the results of sixteen randomized clinical trials were compared. Testosterone was administered in these trials transdermally, orally, or by injection. "Neither short-term nor long-term [replacement therapy] showed significant changes in the four determinants of prostate growth investigated compared with placebo," concluded the authors of this study review.[21]

In the *British Journal of Urology International*, a team of scientists from Germany, Britain, the Netherlands, and the United States did thirty-six months of follow-up with 999 men who had clinically diagnosed hypogonadism. Of those, 750 initiated testosterone replacement therapy (TRT). In the treated men, their mean testosterone levels almost doubled during the study period. When suspected prostate cancer, based on biopsies, was compared between the treated and untreated groups, it was found "the proportion of positive biopsies was nearly identical in men on TRT compared to those not on TRT over the course of the study." This led the scientists to conclude in 2017, "Results support prostate safety of TRT in newly diagnosed men with hypogonadism."[22]

Finally, in a huge 2017 study involving 192,838 men published in the *Journal of Clinical Oncology*, no aggressive prostate cancer risk was observed for men doing replacement therapy. The science team used the National Prostate Cancer Register of Sweden for data in this case-control study. TRT was "significantly associated with more favorable-risk prostate cancer and lower risk of aggressive prostate cancer."[23]

Study coauthor Stacy Loeb of New York University, told *Science-Daily*, "Overall, our study suggests that what is best for men's health is to keep testosterone levels balanced and within a normal range." He further suggested that men whose testosterone levels fall below

350 nanograms per deciliter should consider undertaking replacement therapy.[24]

Is TRT Dangerous to Cardiovascular and Heart Health?

There is scientific evidence accumulating that having a testosterone deficiency is, in and of itself, a significant risk factor for developing cardiovascular disease.

This alert was sounded by four scientists at the Boston University School of Medicine, Department of Biochemistry and Urology, in a 2009 science article. They framed the issue this way: "A considerable body of evidence exists suggesting that androgen deficiency contributes to the onset, progression, or both of cardiovascular disease (CVD)." In other words, the more severe your testosterone deficiency, the greater your risk for developing severe cardiovascular disease.

The reason why a testosterone deficiency may trigger CVD was explained: "Androgen deficiency is associated with increased levels of total cholesterol, low-density lipoprotein, increased production of proinflammatory factors, and increased thickness of the arterial wall and contributes to endothelial dysfunction. Testosterone supplementation restores arterial vasoreactivity, reduces proinflammatory cytokines, total cholesterol, and triglyceride levels, and improves endothelial function but also might reduce high-density lipoprotein levels."[25]

In the *Journal of the American Medical Association Internal Medicine*, a research team described in 2017 how they compared 8,808 men, with an average age of fifty-eight years, who had received testosterone therapy, to 35,527 men, average age of fifty-nine years, who had never received this therapy. Follow-up lasted between three and four years, during which adverse cardiac events were recorded. The results: "Among men with androgen deficiency, dispensed testosterone prescriptions were associated with a lower risk of cardiovascular outcomes" compared to those men never given testosterone therapy.[26]

Scientists from institutions such as the Boston University School of Medicine and the Boston University School of Public Health did an observational study of 656 men, average age of sixty years, who had symptoms of hypogonadism. Half of the men received testosterone undecanoate treatment, 1,000 mg a day. The other group was untreated. Follow-up with both groups occurred over a seven-year period.

The results reported from this study, in 2017, were striking in their support of testosterone therapy improving cardiovascular health: "The estimated reduction in mortality for the T-group was between 66 percent and 92 percent. There were also thirty nonfatal strokes and twenty-six nonfatal myocardial infarctions in the control group and none in the T-treated group. Long-term [testosterone treatment] was well tolerated with excellent adherence suggesting a high level of patient satisfaction. Mortality related to CV [cardiovascular disease] was significantly reduced in the T-group."[27]

Two British scientists, in 2018, examined the scientific study evidence for a relationship between cardiovascular disease and testosterone therapy and concluded, "The weight of evidence from long-term epidemiological studies supports a protective effect as evidenced by a reduction in major adverse cardiovascular events and mortality in studies that have treated men with testosterone deficiency."[28]

So, the weight of scientific evidence points to TRT actually being protection of cardiovascular and heart health, rather than being a risk.[29, 30]

What about a Link to Strokes and Heart Attacks?

After an initial scare in medical circles during the late 1990s, the alleged link between strokes and heart attacks and TRT began to wither away in the face of mounting scientific study evidence.[31] Canadian scientists analyzed all randomized controlled trials on testosterone, from 1980 to 2010, to measure the impact of replacement therapy on exercise capacity and poor clinical outcomes in patients with heart failure.

They found that not only was testosterone therapy "associated with a significant improvement in exercise capacity compared with placebo," but it also happened in these studies without "any significant cardiovascular events." This finding led the study review team to declare, "Testosterone appears to be a promising therapy to improve functional capacity in patients with HF (heart failure)."[32]

By retrospectively examining 83,010 male veterans with documented low total testosterone levels, researchers were able to compare those who had undergone testosterone replacement with those who hadn't, to see the differences in the incidence of stroke, heart attack, and all-cause mortality. Writing of their results in the *European Heart Journal* in 2015, the science team observed how "normalization of TT (total testosterone) levels after TRT (testosterone replacement therapy) was associated with a significant reduction in all-cause mortality, MI (myocardial infarction—heart attack), and stroke."[33]

One leading cause of strokes is atrial fibrillation, a quivering or irregular heartbeat that can trigger blood clots and heart failure. Scientists from the University of Kansas Medical Center assessed a group of 76,639 men with low total testosterone levels and divided them into three groups: one had undergone testosterone replacement resulting in normalization of levels, the second group had replacement therapy without normalization, and the third group received no replacement therapy. It was found that among the first group, in which replacement had normalized total testosterone, they "had significantly lower risk of atrial fibrillation than the other two groups." These results were published in the *Journal of the American Heart Association*, in 2017.[34]

Does TRT Worsen Lower Urinary Tract Symptoms?

Men with moderate to severe lower urinary tract symptoms have traditionally been warned by mainstream physicians to never use testosterone replacement therapy for fear of worsening those symptoms.

To test whether that advice was founded on evidence or just unsubstantiated fear, scientists in the Department of Urology at Northwestern University did a study with 120 men with low testosterone, who received TRT in the form of topical therapy or pellet-based therapy.

These men used TRT for an average of 692 days. Their urinary tract symptoms were assessed using the AUASI (American Urological Association symptom index) both before and after their TRT. Other measures were taken of their PSA (prostate specific antigen) and their testosterone levels.

At the conclusion of the study, the greatest improvement in AU-ASI scores was in men with a PSA greater than 4.0 ng/dL (4.0 and below is considered normal). As the study author wrote in the *Journal of Urology*, "We demonstrate that initiating testosterone replacement therapy in hypogonadal men involves a low risk of worsening lower urinary tract symptoms. In fact, many men experience symptom improvement while changes in prostate specific antigen appear minor."[35]

Further verification of these findings came from scientists in Japan, at Kobe University Graduate School of Medicine, who studied the effects of TRT on sixty men with lower urinary tract symptoms. These men were given 250 mg injections of testosterone every three to four weeks, as a series of measures were taken of their prostate, PSA levels, urinary symptoms including urine volume, erectile function, and both total and free testosterone levels, before and six months after TRT. The result: "This study revealed that TRT appeared to have considerable therapeutic effects on lower urinary tract symptoms, particularly on [urinary] storage symptoms, in men with late-onset hypogonadism."[36]

Finally, in a *European Urology* study review of fourteen clinical trials, involving 2,029 patients, examining whether TRT exacerbated lower urinary tract symptoms, researchers from three U.S. universities concluded in 2016, after contrasting all of the findings, that "TRT treatment does not worsen LUTS (lower urinary tract symptoms) among men with LOH (late onset hypogonadism)."[37]

Is TRT a "Missing Link" in Brain Health?

To reduce your risk of cognitive decline with advancing age, one treatment link that's too often ignored, says Florida urologist and hormone expert Dr. Kenneth Janson, "is the powerful protective effect of hormone optimization, when offered in conjunction with a healthy lifestyle that includes proper exercise and nutrition."

Most of the risk factors for cognitive decline are well known: obesity, diabetes, sleep apnea, hypertension, depression, chronic stress, sedentary lifestyle, prescription and recreational drugs, and chronic use of alcohol. By contrast, maintaining a healthy lifestyle (which includes doing vigorous exercise, mindfulness meditation, learning new skills, and having healthy nutrition) has been demonstrated in studies to create new cells in the hippocampus part of the brain. This is the brain area that processes short-term memories and determines which ones become long-term memories. The process of creating these new cells involves neuroplasticity, a scientific term for the human brain's ability to form new neural connections.

There is evidence that hormone replacement therapy may assist in memory retention and in maintaining the neuroplasticity brain process. Dr. Janson did a before-and-after cognitive analysis of an eighty-eight-year-old male patient of his, who had undergone testosterone optimization.

Using a battery of diagnostic tests, Dr. Janson measured five major brain functions: (1) composite memory, showing how well a person can recognize, remember, and retrieve words and geometric figures; (2) processing speed, measuring how well a person recognizes and processes information; (3) executive function, rating how well a person recognizes rules or navigates rapid decision-making; (4) reaction time; showing how quickly a person can react to simple and increasingly complex directions; and (5) complex attention, measuring the ability to track and respond to information over lengthy periods of time or to perform mental tasks accurately.[38]

Dr. Janson's elderly patient had scored well below average for his age group in all five of these cognitive measures before starting TRT. Sixteen months of hormone replacement therapy later, the elderly gentleman was again given this battery of tests by Dr. Janson. The result: he improved all of his cognitive scores. Executive function and complex attention scores, in particular, improved dramatically above the average for his age group.

Numerous other patients among Dr. Janson's age management clientele recorded similar improvements in brain cognition, during and after hormone optimization. Some of his patients were even in their thirties and forties. More verification of his approach has been seen in study experiments using both human subjects and lab animals, using testosterone and other hormones.[39, 40, 41]

"We now know that we have the potential to live a long life and maintain our quality of life and youthful brain function, until our final days," observed Dr. Janson. "We focus on early intervention and prevention for heart disease, diabetes and other medical conditions, so why don't we become proactive with our brain function?" TRT can help accomplish that goal.

Occasional Odd Side Effects from Testosterone Replacement

Some of the documented—though rare—side effects seen from TRT may actually strike some readers as humorous. These unintended and unexpected consequences, from just a single dose of gel-administered testosterone were seen by U.S. university researchers in two different experiments.

In the first, 243 men were administered either a placebo in a gel or a dose of testosterone in a gel, and then they took a cognition test to measure their decision-making judgment. One question asked was to assess how much a ball costs if the ball and a bat cost $1.10 total, with the bat costing $1 more than the ball. Men administered the dose of testosterone usually answered—incorrectly—that the ball costs ten cents. The correct answer was the ball costs five cents and the bat $1.05.

Why did most of the TRT dose men get the answer wrong within a few hours after being administered the dose? The research team believed that the TRT dose increased confidence that their snap judgments (gut instincts) were correct, which impaired their ability to make rational decisions.[42]

Another unusual effect was observed in a group of men, aged eighteen to fifty-five years, who got either a placebo treatment or a dose of testosterone. They were then asked to choose from among several products, all of which were similar in quality, though one was considered to be more of a luxury brand than the others.

The testosterone group became more prone to choosing the more expensive luxury brand, apparently, so the scientists concluded, because the testosterone increased their desire to make a favorable impression for the purpose of enhancing their status.[43] Other aspects of this phenomenon appear in some men, after they begin TRT, when they impulsively go on buying binges, such as splurging on expensive cars or jewelry to impress women.

An Antidote to Low T We Would *Not* Recommend

When it comes to using "natural" approaches to raising testosterone levels, as an adjunct to TRT or a replacement for it, we certainly wouldn't promote this one. Smoking cigarettes is one of the most noxious and dangerous habits we can think of, responsible for millions of deaths from cancer and heart disease. Yet cigarette smoke, for some unknown reason, has a positive effect on testosterone levels.

A science study published in 2013, assessing the effects of smoking on serum levels of total testosterone, free testosterone, and bioavailable testosterone, found that smokers "had significantly higher total testosterone and free testosterone levels compared to nonsmokers," even after accounting for age, body mass index, triglycerides, and alcohol consumption. More research is needed to determine the biological mechanism for this effect, but there is speculation it is related to one or more of the dozens of chemical components in tobacco smoke, acting as a trigger or protective influence on testosterone production.[44]

Are There Effective Alternatives to TRT?

Throughout this book we've presented a range of "natural" testosterone replacement strategies, from diet and exercise, particularly resistance training, to hormone precursor supplements. Ideally, we would hope that you might couple all of these options together into a cohesive lifestyle intervention program.

We've discussed the large body of scientific research showing the benefits of certain herbs as testosterone-boosting nutrients, as well as certain foods that naturally contain high levels of nutrients like zinc, helpful to testosterone production in the body.

Whether you choose to try natural approaches solely or in collaboration with a testosterone replacement therapy, the goal is for you to take the necessary steps to ensure that the symptoms of andropause no longer limit you from experiencing lifelong quality health. We find ourselves in agreement with the psychotherapist Jed Diamond, who has pointed out how some hormone therapy clinics start a man on hormone replacement therapy as a first resort, when it should be considered a last resort. Proper nutrition, lifestyle, and exercise choices that trigger testosterone levels to rise should be addressed first.

Is DHEA Supplementation Effective in Raising Testosterone?

Its scientific name is Dehydroepiandrosterone, otherwise known as DHEA, another naturally occurring hormone within the human body. It plays a role as a "precursor" (a chemical coming before another chemical, in a process) for androstenedione and androstenediol, which in turn convert to testosterone in the body. Like a row of dominos about to fall, remove one domino and the falling process to completion is impaired.

Though oral supplementation with DHEA remains unregulated by the U.S. Food and Drug Administration, which doesn't consider it to be an anabolic steroid, its use to increase testosterone concentrations has been studied by scientists. The study findings have been mixed and largely inconclusive.

Canadian urologists studied eighty-six men with low testosterone levels by dividing them up into three groups, giving them 50 mg of DHEA twice a day, 80 mg of oral testosterone undecanoate twice daily, or a placebo. The study found testosterone in the DHEA group "increased insignificantly" between the start and finish of the study. Nor was any benefit seen in erectile function.[45]

A similar study done with twenty-four men, average age of sixty-five years, made a comparison of taking 50 mg of DHEA daily for two months to taking a placebo. As reported in the science journal *Clinical Endocrinology*, a modest increase in testosterone was measured in the DHEA group, but it also showed a decrease in LDL cholesterol, the unhealthy kind of cholesterol.[46]

By contrast, a twelve-week study of DHEA supplementation with forty men who routinely exercised, average age of forty-eight years, using 50 mg capsules ingested twice a day, found "DHEA does not independently elicit a statistically significant increase in testosterone levels in healthy adult men." There is some reason to wonder whether a different result would have occurred in sedentary men.[47]

To test the effect of DHEA supplements on sedentary men, scientists writing in the *European Journal of Applied Physiology* in 2013 described how they placed eight sedentary men, average age of forty-nine years, into a DHEA group (50 mg daily) and another eight younger men (average age of twenty-one years) in a placebo-administered group. Both groups did five sessions of cycling exercises and then had their testosterone levels measured. While total testosterone levels dropped for both groups, the DHEA group results demonstrated that "oral DHEA supplementation can elevate free testosterone levels in middle-aged men and prevent it from declining during high-intensity interval training."[48]

What About the Alleged Testosterone "Booster" Supplements?

By some estimates, more than 130 different testosterone "booster" supplement products are being marketed on television, the internet, and other advertising campaigns, making this a $5 billion industry. These products either contain combinations of herbs, vitamins, and minerals or combinations of these mixed with proprietary chemical ingredients. They go by names such as Test RX, TestoGen, Testo Fuel, Nugenix, Prosolution Plus, Testo-Max, and others.

Most of the brands call themselves testosterone "boosters," but this is a bit of a misnomer. These products seek to restore testosterone, bring it back to normal levels, not boost it, since boosting implies increasing it above healthy normal levels, which is what some competitive bodybuilders attempt to do. Some of the supplement brands also claim to "boost" growth hormone (HGH) levels along with testosterone and DHEA. Very few of these products have been subjected to any serious, independent, or authoritative science study scrutiny.

An online review done of testosterone supplements sold on websites like BodyBuilding.com, MensFitness, BodyNutrition, and others, compared their ingredients, based on what their labels identified, to determine whether any of the ingredients had undergone scientific validation as effective in testosterone restoration. Reviews.com concluded that the superior products were the ones containing such ingredients as zinc, magnesium, fenugreek, and long jack (also called tongkat ali), all of which have found some scientific study backing in studies of testosterone support or replacement, as we have detailed in earlier chapters of this book.[49]

But this word of caution is worth noting from the *American Journal of Men's Health*: "Claims and statements of quality insurance found on the packaging [of testosterone booster supplements] are subject to the discretion of the manufacturer. There is no [U.S.] regulatory agency that confirms the accuracy of the information found on the labels, including claims of quality, effectiveness, or ingredients."[50]

Only by religiously reading the product labels and identifying the ingredients, and then determining which have been subjected to scientific study, can you truly begin to learn which products might potentially be beneficial. Otherwise, you are a guinea pig in your own body experiments every time you use one of these "booster" products making unsubstantiated claims.

How to Choose a Hormone Replacement Doctor or Clinic

To begin with, it's important to work only with a physician with the training and experience to determine what is right for you based on your hormone optimization needs. Examine the physician's or clinic's credentials, read reviews of their work and record, and even talk to current patients if you can to gauge their satisfaction levels. Research whether the physician or hormone optimization clinic has been charged with abuse or malpractice by state boards of medicine.

Prescribing any hormone replacement needs to be individualized and based on many factors, including regular follow-up lab studies, dosage adjustments, and clinical follow-up exams. It's probably a good idea to avoid any physician or "hormone optimization" clinic that doesn't prescribe and treat based on your individual physiology and needs.

As you can imagine, adequately managing the administration of bioidentical hormone therapy requires a physician to have additional training in the proper use of such products. Ideally, the physician should perform a detailed initial laboratory evaluation of the patient before initiating any hormone therapy. Then, over time, it's necessary to do ongoing monitoring of hormone levels, to get the best, safest, and most effective use out of these products.

We've pointed out how any use of bioidentical hormones needs to be individualized based on a patient's unique needs. "One size fits all" is definitely not a desirable goal here. Hormone replacement products should not be used until a patient has been carefully evaluated and found to have suboptimal levels and a clinical indication that treatment would be helpful. Once replacement therapy has started, careful long-term monitoring of a patient's condition is important, together with appropriate laboratory follow-up, since your medical condition may change over time.

Should Women Also Consider Testosterone Restoration?

Though testosterone isn't typically prescribed for women (at least by most physicians and clinics, if only because there is still a perception it's a "male-only" hormone), it's important to understand that women also naturally have testosterone in their bodies, just at much lower levels than men. As happens with men, these levels in women decline with age. (The same is also true for men and their estrogen levels, which are lower than in women but decline in much the same way.)

For women, doing testosterone replacement therapy, especially when it is taken together with bioidentical progesterone, has been shown to have a protective anticancer effect on the breast and uterus. Testosterone restoration in women has also been shown to be highly protective to the heart and brain, which happen to be the two primary testosterone receptors in the human body.[51, 52]

The best and most apparent effect of testosterone supplementation in women, however, shows up in improvements to a woman's libido, mood, and energy levels, particularly if the woman is postmenopausal. Let's examine the scientific research evidence.

Scientists associated with three hospitals in Britain did a systematic study review, in 2017, of using transdermal testosterone in postmenopausal women for the treatment of low sexual desire. Seven randomized controlled trials involving 1,350 women who received testosterone patch treatment were included in the analysis.

"The T [testosterone] group had significantly more satisfying sexual episodes, sexual activity, orgasms, desire, significant change in Personal Distress Scale score . . . compared with the placebo group," the science team concluded. There were no major or serious side effects documented from the testosterone treatment, other than rare minor acne and hair growth.[53]

A second study review, conducted in 2018 by scientists in Portugal, analyzed results from eleven studies and found clear evidence of "testosterone's efficacy on global sexual function and improvement of sexual desire in postmenopausal women." No serious adverse effect from its usage was seen.[54]

Since an estimated one-third of all women experience some sexual dysfunction during the course of their lives, making it a common problem, it should be reassuring that women have a safe and reliable treatment option in testosterone, to improve sexual desire and performance.

Can Human Growth Hormone Be Safely Replaced?   **17**

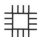

THIS IS A TOPIC THAT DESERVES its own chapter because growth hormone is often overlooked in terms of its importance and its role in the late-life years of both men and women, and because its use in men who have been prescribed it "off-label" remains quite controversial in medical circles. Human growth hormone (HGH), produced by the pituitary gland, is another key human hormone, along with testosterone, that diminishes steadily with age. As HGH levels decline, a variety of musculoskeletal, metabolic, and mental conditions and issues can ensue. As you experience reductions in your skeletal muscle and bone mass strength, for instance, fat retention occurs around your waist, vitality diminishes, cardiovascular risks become heightened, and you may experience an appreciable decline in your mental functions.

Instead of this growth hormone decline, occurring with age and being filed under the label of andropause, where it and its symptoms certainly belong, endocrinologists use another term to define it: somatopause. The *Journal of Clinical Endocrinology and Metabolism* describes it thus: "GH secretion declines by approximately 14% [per decade] from young adult life (20) and some studies suggest that GH secretion may eventually cease in certain elderly subjects."[1]

As occurs with hormone replacement therapy—estrogen in women and testosterone in men—HGH replacement therapy has shown some evidence-backed positive effects in treated persons. It does, however, remain a controversial approach because of medical concerns that have been raised over the years about its long-term safety, particularly as it relates to some forms of cancer.

Origins of Growth Hormone Replacement

Beginning in the 1950s, scientists were injecting children who were short in stature resulting from a growth hormone deficiency with growth hormone extracted from human cadaver pituitary glands. That practice ended when it was discovered that cadavers spread a virulent and incurable brain disorder disease.

As a substitute treatment, recombinant hGH (a molecular cloning process) was developed and then approved by the U.S. Food and Drug Administration. Results in stimulating growth in children were remarkable. In a 2010 assessment of the scientific evidence, it was determined that children receiving the therapy grew 2.7 centimeters a year faster than untreated children.[2]

It wasn't long before physicians began experimenting with growth hormone replacement in adults. They did this by prescribing it "off-label," which means using it to treat a condition other than what the U.S. Food and Drug Administration first approved the drug to treat. In this case, instead of using growth hormone replacement to help children grow faster, a physician might "off-label" it to treat fatigue, obesity, or sexual dysfunction in adults. It is a common and legal practice for a variety of prescription drugs.

"Many people may be surprised to know that the FDA regulates drug approval, not drug prescribing, and doctors are free to prescribe a drug for any reason they think is medically appropriate," G. Caleb Alexander, assistant professor of medicine at the University of Chicago Medical Center, told WebMD. "Off-label use is so common, that virtually every drug is used off-label in some circumstances."[3]

As you can imagine, as anecdotal reports surfaced that growth hormone improved strength, endurance, physical fitness and injury recovery time in adults, professional and amateur athletes began taking advantage of it via injections, to enhance their performance. An entire doping scandal erupted in amateur and professional sports that resulted in the International Olympic Committee adding growth hormone to its list of banned performance-enhancing drugs in 1989. Other professional sports later followed suit.[4]

Though its use remains banned by the World Anti-Doping Agency, detecting growth hormone in random periodic testing has remained a challenge. "Detection of GH doping is challenging for several reasons including identity/similarity of exogenous to endogenous GH, short half-life, complex and fluctuating secretory dynamics of GH, and a very low urinary excretion rate," according to a 2012 science analysis in the journal *Endocrine Reviews*.[5]

While much of the hype surrounding the alleged physical enhancements of growth hormone turned out to be exaggerated, based on the findings of subsequent scientific examinations, there was enough "smoke" to justify the presence of "fire" for growth hormone to find a wider audience among non-athletes, giving rise to physicians emerging to satisfy the demand with off-label prescribing. Those patients seeking growth hormone treatment for the most part don't fall into the category of having pituitary gland impairments resulting in deficient production of growth hormone. Most have bought into the idea that growth hormone replacement is a possible "fountain of youth" elixir, an anti-aging drug to soften or erase many of the symptoms of aging.

Does Growth Hormone Replacement Raise Cancer Risks?

As a theory, or working hypothesis among researchers, the risk of cancer as an outcome of growth hormone replacement therapy came about due to the impact growth hormone and insulin-like growth factor 1 had on promoting cell growth. Evidence emerged from animal and cell (test tube) experiments suggesting that both GH and IGF-1 could be involved with the development of tumors, and as a result, some scientists hypothesized that breast or colon cancer might be triggered in humans.

Early studies in humans had mostly produced mixed results. Some studies indicated an increased cancer risk; other studies did not, or even produced evidence that growth hormone replacement might reduce the risk. In an attempt to add more clarity to the debate, a science review done in 2016 evaluated the findings from nine scientific studies, involving 11,191 participants, to determine the cancer risk in adults who had undergone growth hormone replacement compared to those who had not.

The consensus of these findings, as described in the science journal *Oncotarget* was that "this therapy was associated with the decreased risk of cancer in adults with growth hormone deficiency. Our study suggests that growth hormone replacement therapy could reduce risk of cancer in adults with growth hormone deficiency."[6]

This cancer risk debate over GH may be ongoing. "Over the last 25 years, every few years a paper appears citing a cancer risk, Hodgkin's disease, colon cancer, whatever," said Ron Rosenfeld, professor and chair of Pediatrics at Oregon Health and Science University, in an interview with *Endocrine News*. "And none of those studies has ever been corroborated. So there's a period of alarm, then the pendulum swings the other way. No drug is going to be without risk, and even if you are giving it as a replacement therapy as you do in GHD, we're not entirely mimicking the normal physiology of growth hormone secretion and so we have to always be observant and open to the possibility that there may be adverse effects."[7]

Does It Work to Prevent Frailty in Adults?

While scientists agree that a growth hormone deficiency results in decreased bone mineral density and an increase in a person's risk for fractures, little has been known or agreed about the potential for recombinant growth hormone therapy to treat this problem. In 2014, scientists from Harvard Medical School and other medical institutions sought to address the confusion by reviewing all published science studies investigating growth hormone therapy in connection with bone mineral density, fractures, and resulting frailty in older adults. Their conclusion: "This meta-analysis suggests a beneficial effect of rhGH replacement on bone mineral density in adults with growth hormone deficiency. This effect is affected by gender, age, and treatment duration."[8]

Is It Effective in Treating Obesity in Adults?

A study review of all science research addressing whether recombinant human growth hormone therapy has a positive impact on obesity was conducted in the *Journal of Clinical Endocrinology & Metabolism*, in 2009. "Our metanalysis suggests that rhGH therapy leads to decrease in visceral adiposity and increase in lean body mass as well as beneficial changes in lipid profile in obese adults, without inducing weight loss," the science reviewers determined.[9]

Can It Increase Muscle Strength in Men over Fifty?

To test whether growth hormone administration improves physical capacity in men who don't have a measureable deficiency in growth hormone, scientists writing in the *International Journal of Endocrinology* recruited fourteen healthy men, aged fifty to seventy years, and placed them into two study groups—intervention and placebo. Both groups of study participants had their muscle strength and body composition measured before, during, and after six months of daily leg press, bench press, and other exercises. Those in the group administered growth hormone showed "a statistically significant increase in the leg press responsive muscles" compared to the placebo group. As the study team further reported, "Our study demonstrated an increase in muscle strength in the lower body after GH therapy in healthy men. This finding must be considered and tested in frail older populations."[10]

Natural Solution: Phytochemical Supplementation

There are feasible alternatives to direct HGH replacement that involve plant-based scientific research. This has emerged in experiments with ways to use phytochemicals from various plants to provide safe and effective treatments for HGH loss. Phytochemicals are produced by plants as a defense against diseases and pests, and there are thousands of different types of them.

To give but one example, a March 2018 review of these plant and HGH science findings, conducted by European endocrinologists, identified three isoflavone phytochemicals—genistein, daidzein, and equol—as being promising treatment options. Foods containing these phytochemicals include soy, chickpeas, and fava beans. Soy isoflavone supplements, reported the researchers, are "potentially cheap substances whose easy application shows a number of benefits when it comes to the wide spectrum of ageing symptoms," including HGH loss and its related health conditions.[11]

Natural Solution: Periodic Fasting

Calorie restriction in the form of periodic fasting increases serum growth hormone concentrations, according to science studies, but in some people it may also, ironically, decrease testosterone levels. At the Hippocrates Institute, we suggest all stable people fast at least one day per week.

A study in the *Journal of Clinical Endocrinology & Metabolism* measured blood in test subjects over a twenty-four-hour period, during fasting, and then over a second day, to find that caloric restriction "induced a 5-fold increase in growth hormone production." Though the physiological mechanism for this fasting-induced increase wasn't entirely clear, its appearance led the research team to speculate that periodic fasts over longer periods of time could help to normalize growth hormone levels in men.[12]

By contrast, a 2016 study done over eight weeks, in thirty-four males, found that time-restricted feeding (sixteen hours a day of fasting) resulted in "testosterone and insulin-like growth factor 1 decreasing significantly." Fat mass in the test subjects also decreased.[13]

As a result of these conflicting findings, regular blood testing would probably need to be integrated into any fasting protocol to keep growth hormone increases and testosterone declines in some balance.

Natural Solution: Vigorous Exercise

Much as it happens with testosterone levels, human growth hormone secretions are stimulated by aerobic exercise, most particularly by regular resistance training exercises. To underscore these effects, scientists writing in the *Journal of Applied Physiology* described how they took nine obese men and nine lean men and put them through a daily resistance exercise protocol. The resistance consisted of squat, bench press, leg curls, dumbbell rows, dumbbell shoulder press, and dumbbell step-up exercises, all performed between 7 a.m. and 11 a.m. after twelve hours of overnight fasting. Participants performed three sets of ten repetitions at 85–95 percent of their capacity, since intensity levels below that "would not adequately stimulate a growth hormone response," said the science team. Blood samples were taken pre-exercise, mid-exercise, and immediately post-exercise, and at 50-, 70-, and 110-minute intervals after completion of the exercises.

What the scientists discovered was confirmation of previous studies: "that greater GH (growth hormone) concentrations occur in response to an RE (resistance training) stimulus." Similar positive effects were seen in both the obese and the lean groups of men, as the testing saw "significant" increases in growth hormone after the post-exercise period.[14]

Natural Solution: Royal Jelly

Hundreds of scientific studies have been performed over the past few decades on the medicinal effects in humans of royal jelly, a natural substance that's secreted from glands in the heads of worker bees for nutritional use by the queen bee. Ancient cultures used royal jelly primarily for speeding up wound healing, though it has also been found in recent laboratory analysis to be useful in fighting tumor formation and inflammation and in treating diabetes, hypertension, and high cholesterol. Its chemical composition makes it a rich source of bioactive substances, such as amino acids, B-complex vitamins, and trace minerals.[15]

Still another use is its support of pituitary gland health, triggering growth hormone production by compensating for age-associated decline in pituitary functions. That was the conclusion reached by a team of Japanese scientists in 2009, after testing royal jelly on lab animals.[16]

Two Perspectives on the Safety and Usefulness of GH Treatment

Because aging results in the pituitary gland gradually reducing the amount of growth hormone it produces, human growth hormone treatment therapies have been widely promoted as an anti-aging elixir to maintain health and vitality later in life, and to reverse decreases in bone and muscle mass. Needless to say, the use of these treatments remains controversial, even among age management (or anti-aging) specialists.

Hormone expert and Florida urologist Dr. Kenneth Janson's position on HGH is clearly cautious, as he noted in an interview with our research associate Randall Fitzgerald: "I rarely use it with my patients, for two reasons. First, it is prohibitively expensive; and second, and more importantly, there is still a lot we do not know about the long-term use of HGH (such as possible cancer risk, etc.). Though in the short term, its use doesn't appear to increase cancer risks, the jury is still out on the longer-term effects."

"On the other hand, in patients that have a documented lab-proven adult onset growth hormone deficiency, and who have failed other forms of therapy, HGH can be highly effective. Under those circumstances, I would be open-minded about using it carefully, but only if the patient understands the potential long-term risks, as well as the potential benefits. There are also definite benefits of HGH in specific groups of patients, with cardiovascular disease, and other serious health issues as well."[17, 18, 19]

A rather different view comes from James Forsythe, an oncologist who uses growth hormone replacement treatments in his clinic and wrote a book about it, *Anti-Aging Cures: Life Changing Secrets to Reverse the Effects of Aging*. The foreword was written by Suzanne Somers, the actress and author of more than twenty books, who is known as the face of anti-aging medicine and an outspoken advocate for bioidentical hormone replacement therapy in both women and men.

In his book, Dr. Forsythe calls HGH the "Master Hormone" that "orchestrates all of endocrine hormone functions in the body, such as your sex hormones." He describes two approaches to restoring growth hormone in the body—using injectable growth hormone replacement or noninvasive "biostimulators" such as royal jelly, with what they have in common being "their ability to change your biochemistry through the new science of bioidentical blueprinting."[20]

Once his patients begin receiving growth hormone replacement, Dr. Forsythe claims they experience a range of "age-reversal effects": skin tightening and wrinkle disappearance, bone density improvement, heightened energy, memory and mental clarity sharpening, more consistent sleep quality, immune system strengthening, metabolism going up and visceral fat disappearing, hair thinning stopping, and libido and sexual performance showing dramatic improvement.

Until scientists figure out how to deliver HGH via slow-release pellets or capsules, HGH must be injected because the human digestive system cannot absorb it without breaking it down until it's useless before it reaches the liver. As a result, HGH injections need to be administered three to six times a week, at a cost that Dr. Forsythe estimated (when his book was published in 2011) to be up to $400–$600 per month. Insurance coverage will pay only if you have AIDS wasting condition, adult short bowel syndrome, or a continuation of treatment of childhood growth hormone deficiency.

As for claims that HGH injections over time can cause side effects such as diabetes, carpal tunnel syndrome, joint pain, or extended bellies, Dr. Forsythe declared that none of his patients at his Century Wellness Clinic have exhibited any of these alleged symptoms.[21]

Andropause + Menopause = Couplepause   18

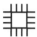

E ARLIER IN THIS BOOK, we introduced you to the term *Irrita-ble Male Syndrome* (IMS), first coined in 2002 by Dr. Gerald A. Lincoln, a Scottish human reproductive sciences researcher, based on his observations of men with low testosterone exhibiting a slew of interconnected psychological conditions: irritability, anxiety, lethargy, and depression. "Men experiencing IMS can change, seemingly overnight, from peaceful to agitated, from loving to mean, from contented to discontented," wrote psychotherapist Jed Diamond, in his book about the phenomenon.[1] As a result of the fear and confusion these men feel, they may withdraw from close relationships, even end a marriage while pursuing younger women, in order to feel less trapped and more in control of their life. Their IMS behaviors may include chronic criticism of others, expressing contempt or mockery, denying responsibility for what is happening, and refusing to tell the truth about what they are feeling. In extreme cases, these behaviors can even lead to violence against their partners. Some therapists have noted how alcohol and drug use may increase and dependence on these substances intensify as a man undergoes andropause, with the symptoms of anger and frustration accompanying it.

Men who are in denial about being in andropause have a personal war zone going on within them. The man is thinking to himself, "What happened to me? I was known for my brilliance, and now I can't think straight. I used to be virile, and now I've lost it." This attitudinal atmosphere is sensed by women because they reside more in empathy and compassion. As a result, they are more affected by andropause than men ever suspect. We know because women tell us all the time how sad they are about losing the intimacy they once shared with their partner.

As a culture, we need to educate men that andropause isn't a sign of weakness and it's possible to experience healthy aging if they change their lifestyle. By adopting a healthier diet and regular exercise, along with supplements (such as full-spectrum liquid ginseng and flower pollen) and properly prescribed bioidentical hormones, all of these elements working together can bring about a radical shift back to some semblance of youth.

Convincing a man to seek help can be the most serious challenge. Let's imagine we have an amenable man, one who isn't in denial. We recommend counseling with a psychotherapist who can explain why he feels angry, why his muscles are aching, and why his sleep patterns are disrupted. These are symptoms of normal hormonal decline, but there is something that can be done about the condition.

Many women, when they turn fifty or sixty years of age and start to have memory and sleep problems, have learned to recognize the symptoms of menopause and get themselves on bioidentical hormones. Most men never receive that education or develop that awareness. When the woman's condition improves and their sexuality returns, oftentimes the husband freaks out. If the man can overcome his denial about his own hormonal decline, it's an opening for him to undertake his own treatment and clean up his own act, getting inspiration from the woman's visible radical improvement as a result of taking bioidentical hormone therapy.

Andropause can be a disorienting crisis of identity. Novelist Tim Lott, writing in Britain's *Daily Mail* newspaper, described what befell a couple he knew, Mike and Sally, both in their early fifties, who had been married for two decades. Mike unexpectedly left their marriage, telling Sally he felt trapped and unhappy; he no longer thought he loved her. There was no other woman in his life or any seemingly rational explanation for his abrupt departure. Sally started researching male midlife depression on the internet and came across a website describing a condition called male menopause. "Every single element of his behavior—from his mood swings to his bizarre denial of any happy past together—was laid out in bullet points as a symptom of the so-called 'andropause.'" Sally learned that what afflicted her husband "was not just a mid-life crisis, but could be a genuine medical syndrome."[2]

What did Sally do with this newfound knowledge? "Far from condemning him for his seemingly selfish and irrational mid-life crisis, she now faced the question: should she have sympathy for a possible hormone imbalance over which he had no more control than any woman going through menopause?" For Sally, along with many women in similar circumstances, compassion won out over retribution.

To maintain a solid loving relationship, you both want to be on the same page, sharing the energy and vitality to remain active together and love together. Men need to face up and answer several questions. Don't you want to be there for your wife? Don't you want to be in sync again? Do you want to be a loser or a winner? Some guys are so shallow and frightened and immature, they would never admit they have a problem. That makes the women in their life sad and understandably frustrated.

Psychotherapist Diamond proposed a dozen actions a caring partner can take to assist a man who is in denial about having IMS and being in andropause: don't try to push him into changing; ask what his denial is triggering in you; keep a focus on taking care of yourself; realize you are not the target of his moods; listen to how he feels; let him know you are open to listening; walk and talk with him; let him know that you care; get support from others; seek a counselor if necessary; be firm with him; and, most especially, don't give up.

Hormonal Imbalance Consequences for a Couple

Have you ever been in a dating relationship, or in a marriage, and the two of you find yourselves going through hormone imbalances at the same time? You may not have even consciously realized it at the time, though the symptoms were present for everyone to see.

If that's been your experience, or if you have observed this phenomenon in another couple, you understand how it can further complicate the set of challenges every couple normally faces in their relational health. When menopause in a woman occurs simultaneously with andropause in a man, it can become what some endocrinologists and sex therapists refer to as "couplepause," resulting in the potential for relationship disharmony and shared sexual dysfunction.

Menopause symptoms in women, such as hot flashes, mood changes, and loss of libido, when matched with symptoms of andropause in men, most typically irritability, fatigue, and loss of sexual function, can make it seem like the relationship is undergoing a disturbing transition for the worse. This is especially true if the underlying hormonal imbalances are left untreated by either partner.

We have observed over the decades, among guests at our Hippocrates Health Institute in Florida, that when a hormonal decline occurs in one partner, in short order we start to see a decline occurring in the other partner. We suspect that pheromones (chemicals secreted as part of sexual attraction) play a role in the way this subtle partner-to-partner communication happens. This pheromone connection may also result in the hormonal symptoms seen in one partner being mirrored and intensified in the other.

When a male loses his virility due to hormonal decline, sometimes the woman in his life no longer feels as useful or attractive as their sexual connection evaporates. The less sex they have, as a result, the more they lose interest in it, so there is a natural relationship rhythm that's disrupted when hormones are unbalanced. (For a more in-depth guide, you might read our book, 7 *Keys to Lifelong Sexual Vitality*.)

Men lose interest in sex, oftentimes due to sexual dysfunction, decades before women because of the natural biological clock. But social norms have traditionally dictated that men are supposed to be virile (or act virile) in all life ages. So there is a dance going on between social norms and biology. It's like a dark Shakespearean play. Most cultures are geared to treat men as the embodiment of strength, control and virility; anything less is seen as a symptom of weakness. These social norms imposed on men, such as their gray hair and wrinkles being regarded as "distinguished" contrast with women historically not being viewed this way in the last quarter of life.

The conversation we hear among our health care guests on a weekly basis is an angry one in which the man is frustrated and doesn't feel like satisfying his intimacy role in the relationship, and the woman feels bad and pretends she doesn't care, but she does care because she's frustrated, too. There is rarely a healthy conversation surrounding hormonal imbalances, and most people don't seem to realize there are readily available treatment options.

We also have considerable personal experience working with men who exhibit symptoms of irritable male syndrome. Mary and Charles are a good example (we changed their names to protect their privacy). Both are in their fifties, and she told us they had a great marriage for twenty-eight years, but seven years ago he started becoming highly critical of her. She would always ask him when he came home from work how his day had been, and he began to snap at her with irritability. He wasn't communicative anymore. First thing at night he switched off the light as a sign of sexual disinterest. She thought he was having an affair, which further strained their relationship.

Finally, their son, who had been experiencing erectile dysfunction and found relief using bioidentical hormones at our health institute, referred his father to us. Charles cleaned up his diet and went on testosterone hormone therapy. By the third week of treatment, he was feeling and acting normal again. Mary got her husband back. He is a living testament to how the biochemistry of hormones can be an indicator of one's emotional state.

Counselor Dennis Marasco laid out the options a couple often faces when trying to decide their best course of action:

> If this couple goes to a therapist, the therapist might work on strengthening their communication. If they were to go to a medical doctor, he or she might recommend testosterone supplementation. If instead, they went to see a psychiatrist, he or she might recommend an antidepressant. If they had gone to a nutritionist, a focus on a healthy diet would have likely been suggested. Finally, a fitness expert would have advised the couple to engage in cardio and strengthening exercises. Maybe many of these recommendations would be the combined treatment of choice to help get this couple back on track.[3]

Hormone Treatment Needs to Involve Both Partners

When a couple goes through hormonal changes at the same time, their challenge isn't only the need to be helpful and compassionate and sensitive to each other's needs. They need to adjust to psychological changes that affect their ability to effectively resolve personal conflict. They must also support each other in taking treatment steps to reestablish a healthy hormonal balance.

"Both members of a couple may experience age-related changes concurrently and interdependently," wrote medical specialists in the journal *Sexual Medicine Review*. "In such cases, it is unhelpful, and sometimes detrimental, to treat the symptoms for only one member of the couple without treating the other."[4] To illustrate, if the male partner in the relationship receives treatment with hormone replacement therapy, and the other partner doesn't receive corresponding estrogen replacement treatment and needs it, the untreated partner can actually experience psychological mini-traumas, including depression. Or if one partner regains his or her libido as a result of hormone replacement therapy, and the other doesn't feel a sexual rebound, that could seed frustration and even philandering into the relationship.

Educating and treating both partners simultaneously can soften the impacts of midlife hormone decline by providing a mutual support system to enhance the effectiveness of the treatment protocols. In a 2018 *Sexual Medicine Review* article, it was pointed out how there is a "need for a new diagnostic and therapeutic paradigm that addresses the sexual health needs of the aging couple as a whole rather than treating the individual patient in isolation. Taking a couple-oriented approach to evaluate and manage couplepause in the latter half of life can dramatically and simultaneously help both members of the couple to improve sexual satisfaction and intimacy."

The science paper further stated, "Symptoms in one partner may worsen the other partner's symptoms. Therefore, by addressing the sexual health needs of a patient without considering the potential impact on or contributions of the partner's health, clinicians are not fulfilling the real-life needs of older couples. A couples-oriented approach to treating sexual dysfunction in the climacteric couple has not been widely adopted, nor has it been used systematically to understand how sexual dysfunction of the aging male can amplify the sexual dysfunction of the aging female partner and vice versa. Male and female sexual symptoms are frequently multiplicative rather than additive, such that symptoms in one partner may exacerbate symptoms in the other."

Scientific studies have supported how this cross-influence phenomenon occurs. For example, a survey of ninety-six New Zealand women whose partners had erectile dysfunction found that half of the women also had sexual dysfunction, and many of them attributed their condition "exclusively to their partner's ED." When their partner's ED was treated, most of these women experienced improved sexual function.[5]

Be Aware of Your Impact on Future Generations

In our fifty years of doing clinical work, we've seen a radical shift in the age at which menopause and andropause begins. When we began our work, men and women were usually in their fifties when the hormonal changes made an appearance with visible symptoms. Over the past decade or so, the average age of onset for hormonal imbalance has dropped into the low forties. Sometimes we see it occurring even in a person's thirties.

Andrew and Sally characterize this phenomenon. She is a physician, now in her mid-fifties; he is a businessman in his early fifties. They started coming to see us about ten years ago, when she was struggling emotionally and physically with menopause in her early forties. As Sally got treatment, we saw her husband going through what he believed was a midlife crisis. He thought his symptoms were just a sign of getting old. He never imagined he could be going through the male equivalent of what his wife was going through.

When we suggested to Andrew that he take a hormone test, his response was "No, that's for women." After much persuasion, he agreed to have his hormone levels checked, and it turned out that he had almost nonexistent testosterone, which was shocking given his relatively young age. He went on testosterone replacement therapy, supplemented with ginseng, and though he didn't rebound as quickly as his wife, he did eventually undergo a significant reduction in all his andropause symptoms.

We are now aware of a new approach to take with andropausal men who are still desirous of fathering children. It goes beyond the personal self-interest appeal that usually motivates men to seek treatment.

In a series of three research studies that shook the foundations of human biology when they were published in *The Lancet* medical journal, in 2018 a concept was introduced called "pre-conception health." It came from a study conducted by an international research team from universities and hospitals in Britain, Australia, South Africa, the Netherlands, and India. They revealed how the health of both men and women before a child is conceived has a more profound impact on the lifelong mental and physical condition of their offspring than anyone previously knew or suspected.

During the three- to six-month period before a couple conceives, the couple's risk factors connected to their lifestyle habits, dietary choices, body weight, metabolism, and more is like a formula that's ready to be mixed at conception to create a lifetime genetic health legacy for their future children. Research data had previously supported the woman's role in this process, particularly if she was obese, which made the child more susceptible to obesity. But this new research highlighted the critical role of a father's lifestyle and hormonal health in influencing the inherited chronic disease state of his offspring.[6, 7, 8]

A follow-up 2019 study by a separate research team, published in the *Journal of Endocrinology*, focused on environmental exposure influences and male diet and health status, which interact to "affect offspring growth and metabolism leading to increased risk for cardio-metabolic and neurological disease in later life."[9]

As men start manifesting the symptoms of andropause at younger and younger ages, and as women's childbearing years are stretched by advances in reproductive science, male hormonal imbalances play an increasing and possibly toxic role in the preconception risk factors that must be taken into account to protect a child's developmental health.

Prevention strategies must now encompass educating men not only about how hormonal imbalances undermine their own health but also about how they can also pass these genetic markers on to their children, tainting their health legacy. Our evolution as a species may depend on how seriously prospective parents take these disturbing scientific findings and how aggressively they embrace treatment strategies for keeping human health and hormones in balance.

Notes

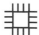

Introduction

1. Rowan Pelling, "Watching the Male Menopause in Action Isn't Pretty," *The Telegraph*, July 30, 2015, https://www.telegraph.co.uk/men/active/mens-health/11774259/Watching-the-male-menopause-in-action-isnt-pretty.html (accessed 2/16/19).

2. G. Jakiel et al., "Andropause—State of the Art 2015 and Review of Selected Aspects," *Menopause Review*, March 2015.

3. Carol Bradley Bursack, "Andropause: A Taboo Topic for Many Men," AgingCare.com, https://www.agingcare.com/articles/andropause-a-taboo-topic-for-many-men-197063.htm (accessed 2/4/19).

4. T. G. Travison et al., "A Population-Level Decline in Serum Testosterone Levels in American Men," *Journal of Clinical Endocrinology & Metabolism*, January 2007.

Chapter One: Give Yourself This Andropause Assessment

1. G. Jakiel et al., "Andropause—State of the Art 2015 and Review of Selected Aspects," *Menopause Review*, March 2015.

2. J. E. Morley et al., "Validation of a Screening Questionnaire for Androgen Deficiency in Aging Males," *Metabolism*, 2000.

3. O. Mohammed et al., "The Quantitative ADAM Questionnaire: A New Tool in Quantifying the Severity of Hypogonadism," *International Journal of Impotence Research*, January 2010.

4. C. Lee et al., "The Prevalence and Correlates of the Positive Androgen Deficiency in the Aging Male (ADAM) Questionnaire among Psychiatric Outpatients: A Cross-Sectional Survey of 176 Men in a General Hospital in Taiwan," *Neuropsychiatric Disease Treatment*, January 2015.

5. N. N. Stone et al., "Male Androgen Deficiency Syndrome Screening Questionnaire: A Simplified Instrument to Identify Testosterone-Deficient Men," *Journal of Men's Health*, April 2014.

Chapter Two: Untreated Andropause Undermines Male Health

1. Lawrence D. Komer, "Andropause: Roy's Story," Komer Health Centre, http://komer-womens-health.com/male-menopause/ (accessed 2/16/19).

2. Tom Nikkola, "Irritable Male Syndrome, Andropause, and Reclaiming Your Manhood," *TomNikkola Newsletter*, https://tomnikkola.com/irritable-male-syndrome-andropause-manhood/ (accessed 2/16/19).

3. Winifred Cutler, *Love Cycles: The Science of Intimacy* (New York: Random House, 1995).

4. Jed Diamond, "What Your Doctor Won't Tell You about Male Hormonal Cycles," GoodTherapy.org. October 9, 2012, https://www.goodtherapy.org/blog/male-hormonal-cycles-andropause-1009127 (accessed 2/16/19).

5. C. U. Eziefula et al., "You Know I've Joined Your Club . . . I'm in the Hot Flush Boy: A Qualitative Exploration of Hot Flashes and Night Sweats in Men Undergoing Androgen Deprivation Therapy for Prostate Cancer," *Psycho-oncology*, December 2013.

6. C. Y. Chen et al., "The Correlation between Emotional Distress and Aging Males' Symptoms at a Psychiatric Outpatient Clinic: Sexual Dysfunction as a Distinguishing Characteristic between Andropause and Anxiety/Depression in Aging Men," *Clinical Interventions in Aging*, 2013.

7. S. Rohrmann et al., "Serum Estrogen, but Not Testosterone, Levels Differ between Black and White Men in a Nationally Representative Sample of Americans," *Journal of Clinical & Endocrinology Metabolism*, July 2007.

8. D. S. Lopez, "Racial/Ethnic Differences in Serum Sex Steroid Hormone Concentrations in US Adolescent Males," *Cancer Causes Control*, April 2013.

9. H. Hu et al., "Racial Differences in Age-Related Variations of Testosterone Levels among US Males: Potential Implications for Prostate Cancer and Personalized Medication," *J Racial Ethn Health Disparities*, March 2015.

.

10. A. M. Traish et al., "The Dark Side of Testosterone Deficiency: III. Cardiovascular Disease," *Journal of Andrology*, September–October 2009.

11. A. M. Traish et al., "The Dark Side of Testosterone Deficiency: II. Type 2 Diabetes and Insulin Resistance," *Journal of Andrology*, January–February 2009.

12. E. R. Schwarz et al., "Andropause and the Development of Cardiovascular Diseases Presentation—More Than an Epi-Phenomenon," *J Geratr Cardiol*, March 2011.

13. M. M. Shores et al., "Increased Incidence of Diagnosed Depressive Illness in Hypogonadal Older Men," *Arch Gen Psychiatry*, February 2004.

14. J. Zhang et al., "Both Total Testosterone and Sex Hormone–Binding Globulin Are Independent Risk Factors for Metabolic Syndrome: Results from Fangchenggang Area Male Health and Examination Survey in China," *Diabetes Metab Res. Rev.*, July 2013.

15. G. A. Laughlin et al., "Low Serum Testosterone and Mortality in Older Men," *J Clin Endocrinol Metab*, January 2008.

16. S. R. Pye et al., "Late-Onset Hypogonadism and Mortality in Aging Men," *J Clin Endocrinol Metab*, April 2014.

17. V. Jaruvongvanich et al., "Testosterone, Sex Hormone–Binding Globulin and Nonalcoholic Fatty Liver Disease: A Systematic Review and Meta-Analysis," *Ann Hepatol*, May 2017.

18. B. B. Yeap et al., "In Older Men, Higher Plasma Testosterone or Dihydrotestosterone Is an Independent Predictor for Reduced Incidence of Stroke but Not Myocardial Infarction," *J Clin Endocrinol Metab*, December 2014.

19. E. L. Ding et al., "Sex Differences of Endogenous Sex Hormones and Risk of Type 2 Diabetes: A Systematic Review and Meta-Analysis," *JAMA*, March 2006.

Chapter Three: Lifestyle Choices and Toxins Accelerate Aging

1. R. Hauser et al., "Male Reproductive Disorders, Diseases, and Costs of Exposure to Endocrine-Disrupting Chemicals in the European Union," *J Clin Endocrinol Metab*, April 2015.

2. N. M. Grindler et al., "Persistent Organic Pollutants and Early Menopause in U.S. Women," *PLOS One*, January 2015.

3. O. Yang et al., "Endocrine-Disrupting Chemicals: Review of Toxicological Mechanisms Using Molecular Pathway Analysis," *J Cancer Prev*, March 2015.

4. L. M. Caronia et al., "Abrupt Decrease in Serum Testosterone Levels after an Oral Glucose Load in Men: Implications for Screening for Hypogonadism," *Clin Endocrinol*, February 2013.

5. "Too Much Sugar Turns Off Gene That Controls Effects of Sex Steroids," *ScienceDaily*, November 21, 2007.

6. L. Chen et al., "Sugar-Sweetened Beverage Intake and Serum Testosterone Levels in Adult Males 20-39 Years Old in the United States," *Reprod Biol Endocrinol*, June 2018.

7. Samuel Epstein and Randall Fitzgerald, *Toxic Beauty: How Cosmetics and Personal-Care Products Endanger Your Health* (Dallas, TX: Benbella, 2009).

8. J. Chen et al., "Antiandrogenic Properties of Parabens and Other Phenolic Containing Small Molecules in Personal Care Products," *Toxicology & Applied Pharmacology*, June 2017.

9. R. J. Witorsch et al., "Personal Care Products and Endocrine Disruption: A Critical Review of the Literature," *Crit Rev. Toxicol*, November 2010.

10. N. Bluthgen, "Effects of the UV Filter Benzophenone-3 (oxybenzone) at Low Concentrations in Zebrafish," *Toxicol Appl Pharmacol*, September 2012.

11. H. R. Contreras et al., "Testosterone Production and Spermatogenic Damage Induced by Organophosphorate Pesticides," *Biocell*, December 30, 2006.

12. F. Orton et al., "Widely Used Pesticides with Previously Unknown Endocrine Activity Revealed as in Vitro Antiandrogens," *Environ Health Perspect*, June 2011.

13. P. Gaudriault et al., "Endocrine Disruption in Human Fetal Testis Explants by Individual and Combined Exposures to Selected Pharmaceuticals, Pesticides, and Environmental Pollutants," *Environ Health Perspect*, August 2017.

14. S. Mediakovic et al., "Effect of Nonpersistent Pesticides on Estrogen Receptor, Androgen Receptor, and Aryl Hydrocarbon Receptor," *Environ Toxicol*, October 2014.

15. C. D. Fryar et al., "Fast Food Consumption among Adults in the United States, 2013-2016," NCHS Data Brief No. 322, October 2018.

16. A. R. Zota et al., "Recent Fast Food Consumption and Bisphenol A and Phtyalates Exposures among the U.S. Population in NHANES, 2003-2010," *Environ Health Perspect*, October 2016.

17. J. R. Varshavsky et al., "Dietary Sources of Cumulative Phthalates Exposure among the U.S. General Population in NHANES 2005-2014," *Environ Int*, June 2018.

18. D. Armanini et al., "Licorice Consumption and Serum Testosterone in Healthy Man," *Exp Clin Endocrinol Diabetes*, September 2003.

19. L. Trasande et al., "Association of Exposure to Di-2-Ethylhex-ylphthalate Replacements with Increased Blood Pressure in Children and Adolescents," *Hypertension*, July 2015.

20. K. Watanabe et al., "Marijuana Extracts Possess the Effects Like the Endocrine Disrupting Chemicals," *Toxicology*, January 2005.

21. J. D. Meeker et al., "House Dust Concentrations of Organophosphate Flame Retardants in Relation to Hormone Levels and Semen Quality Parameters," *Environ Health Perspect*, March 2010.

22. W. J. Crinnion, "Sauna as a Valuable Clinical Tool for Cardiovascular, Autoimmune, Toxicant-Induced and Other Chronic Health Problems," *Altern Med Rev.*, September 2011.

23. W. Crinnion, "Components of Practical Clinical Detox Programs—Sauna as a Therapeutic Tool," *Altern Ther Health Med*, March-April 2007.

24. M. L. Hannuksela et al., "Benefits and Risks of Sauna Bathing," *Am J Med*, February 2001.

25. A. Masuda et al., "The Effects of Repeated Thermal Therapy for Two Patients with Chronic Fatigue Syndrome," *J Psychosom Res*, April 2005.

26. S. Myhill et al., "Targeting Mitochrondrial Dysfunction in the Treatment of Myalgic Encephalomyelitis/Chronic Fatigue Syndrome—a Clinical Audit," *Int J Clin Exp Med*, 2013.

27. M. Sobajima et al., "Waon Therapy Improves Quality of Life as Well as Cardiac Function and Exercise Capacity in Patients with Chronic Heart Failure," *Int Heart J*, 2015.

Chapter Four: Lifting Brain "Fog"

1. S. J. Fuller et al., "Androgens in the Etiology of Alzheimer's Disease in Aging Men and Possible Therapeutic Interventions," *J Alzheimer's Dis*, September 2007.

2. A. H. Ford et al., "Sex Hormones and Incident Dementia in Older Men: The Health in Men Study," *Psychoneuroedocrinology*, September 2018.

3. S. D. Moffat et al., "Longitudinal Assessment of Serum Free Testosterone Concentration Predicts Memory Performance and Cognitive Status in Elderly Men," *J Clin Endcrinol Metab*, November 2002.

4. R. H. Matousek and B. B. Sherwin, "Sex Steroid Hormones and Cognitive Functioning in Healthy, Older Men," *Horm Behav*, March 2010.

5. J. W. Miller et al., "Vitamin D Status and Rates of Cognitive Decline in a Multiethnic Cohort of Older Adults," *JAMA Neurol*, November 2015.

6. S. L. Risacher et al., "Association between Anticholinergic Medication Use and Cognition, Brain Metabolism, and Brain Atrophy in Cognitively Normal Older Adults," *JAMA-Neurology*, April 2016.

7. K. Richardson et al., "Anticolinergic Drugs and Risk of Dementia: Case-Control Study," *BMJ*, April 2018.

8. J. A. Blumenthal et al., "Lifestyle and Neurocognition in Older Adults with Cognitive Impairments: A Randomized Trial," *Neurology*, December 2018.

9. K. Reiter, "Improved Cardiorespiratory Fitness Is Associated with Increased Cortical Thickness in Mild Cognitive Impairment," *Journal of the International Neuropsychological Society*, 2015.

10. Y. Gu et al., "Mediterranean Diet and Brain Structure in a Multiethnic Elderly Cohort," *Neurology*, October 2015.

11. R. J. Hardman et al., "Adherence to a Mediterranean-Style Diet and Effects on Cognition in Adults: A Qualitative Evaluation and Systematic Review of Longitudinal and Prospective Trials," *Front Nutr.*, July 2016.

12. M. C. Morris et al., "MIND Diet Slows Cognitive Decline with Aging," *Alzheimers Dement*, September 2015.

13. S. L. Gardener and S. R. Rainey-Smith, "The Role of Nutrition in Cognitive Function and Brain Ageing in the Elderly," *Curr Nutr Rep*, September 2018.

14. P. Malinowski et al., "Mindful Aging: The Effects of Regular Brief Mindfulness Practice on Electrophysiological Markers of Cognitive and Affective Processing in Older Adults," *Mindfulness*, December 2015.

15. G. Liu et al., "Efficacy and Safety of MMFS-01, a Synapse Density Enhancer, for Treating Cognitive Impairment in Older Adults: A Randomized, Double-Blind, Placebo-Controlled Trial," *J Alzheimers Dis*, 2016.

16. J. T. Hua et al., "Effects of Testosterone Therapy on Cognitive Function in Aging: A Systematic Review," *Cogn Behav Neurol*, September 2016.

17. M. M. Cherrier et al., "Testosterone Supplementation Improves Spatial and Verbal Memory in Healthy Older Men," *Neurology*, July 2001.

18. E. J. Wahjoepramono et al., "The Effects of Testosterone Supplementation on Cognitive Functioning in Older Men," *CNS Neurol Disord Drug Targets*, 2016.

Chapter Five: Handling Depression and Mood Changes

1. G. A. Lincoln, "The Irritable Male Syndrome," *Reprod Fertil Dev*, 2001.

2. L. Sher, "Low Testosterone Levels May Be Associated with Suicidal Behavior in older Men while High Testosterone Levels May Be Related to Suicidal Behavior in Adolescents and Young Adults: A Hypothesis," *Int J Adolesc Med Health*, 2013.

3. L. Sher, "Both High and Low Testosterone Levels May Play a Role in Suicidal Behavior in Adolescent, Young, Middle-Age, and Older Men: A Hypothesis," *Int J Adolesc Med Health*, June 2016.

4. S. Khosravi et al., "Are Andropause Symptoms Related to Depression?" *Aging Clin Exp Res*, December 2015.

5. M. Rabijewski et al., "Hormonal Determinants of the Severity of Andropausal and Depressive Symptoms in Middle-Aged and Elderly Men with Prediabetes," *Clin Interv Aging*, August 2015.

6. M. A. Khusid et al., "The Emerging Role of Mindfulness Meditation as Effective Self-Management Strategy, Part 1: Clinical Implications for Depression, Post-Traumatic Stress Disorder, and Anxiety," *Mil Med*, September 2016.

7. S. Kvam et al., "Exercise as a Treatment for Depression: A Meta-analysis," *J Affect Disord*, September 2016.

8. P. J. Carek et al., "Exercise for the Treatment of Depression and Anxiety," *Int J Psychiatry Med*, 2011.

9. S. A. Saeed et al., "Exercise, Yoga, and Meditation for Depressive and Anxiety Disorders," *Am Fam Physician*, April 2010.

10. "What the Science Says about the Effectiveness of St. John's Wort for Depression," National Center for Complementary and Integrative Health, https://nccih.nih.gov/health/stjohnswort/sjw-and-depression.htm.

11. M. Molendijk et al., "Diet Quality and Depression Risk: A Systematic Review and Dose-Response Meta-Analysis of Prospective Studies," *J Affective Disord*, January 2018.

12. L. Ye et al., "Dietary Patterns and Depression Risk: A Meta-analysis," *Psychiatry Research*, July 2017.

13. M. Lucas et al., "Inflammatory Dietary Pattern and Risk of Depression among Women," *Brain, Behavior, and Immunity*, February 2014.

14. R. K. Sripada et al., "DHEA Enhances Emotion Regulation Neurocircuits and Modulates Memory for Emotional Stimuli," *Neuropsychopharmacology*, August 2013.

15. J. McHenry et al., "Sex Differences in Anxiety and Depression: Role of Testosterone," *Front Neuroendocrinol*, January 2014.

16. S. N. Seidman "Normative Hypogonadism and Depression: Does 'Andropause' Exist?" *Int J Impotence Res*, 2006.

Chapter Six: Combating Bone and Joint Degeneration

1. M. Lashkari et al., "Association of Serum Testosterone and Dehydro-epiandrosterone Sulfate with Rheumatoid Arthritis: A Case Control Study," *Electron Physician*, March 2018.

2. M. Pikwer et al., "Association between Testosterone Levels and Risk of Future Rheumatoid Arthritis in Men: A Population-Based Case-Control Study," *Ann Rheum Dis*, March 2014.

3. M. Janiszewska et al., "Men's Knowledge about Osteoporosis and Its Risk Factors," *Prz Menopauzalny*, November 2016.

4. G. Golds et al., "Male Hypogonadism and Osteoporosis: The Effects, Clinical Consequences, and Treatment of Testosterone Deficiency in Bone Health," *Int J Endocrinol*, 2017.

5. R. A. Adler "Management of Osteoporosis in Men on Androgen Deprivation Therapy," *Maturitas*, February 2011.

6. C. J. Paller et al., "Relationship of Sex Steroid Hormones with Bone Mineral Density (BMD) in a Nationally Representative Sample of Men," *Clin Endocrinol*, January 2009.

7. M. Yimam et al., "UP1306, a Botanical Compositions with Analgesic and Anti-Inflammatory Effect," *Pharmacognosy Res*, July–September 2016.

8. M. Yimam et al., "A Botanical Composition Mitigates Cartilage Degradations and Pain Sensitivity in Osteoarthritis Disease Model," *J Med Food*, June 2017.

9. D. S. Kalman and S. J. Hewlings, "The Effects of *Morus alba* and *Acacia catechu* on Quality of Life and Overall Function in Adults with Osteoarthritis of the Knee," *J Nutr Metab*, 2017.

10. T. H. Wong et al., "Effects of 25-hydroxyvitamin D and Vitamin D-binding Protein on Bone Mineral Density and Disease Activity in Malaysian Patients with Rheumatoid Arthritis," *Int J Rheum Dis*, May 2018.

11. S. M. Alibhai et al., "Changes in Bone Mineral Density in Men Starting Androgen Deprivation Therapy and the Protective Role of Vitamin D," *Osteoporos Int*, October 2013.

12. S. E. Borst et al., "Musculoskeletal and Prostate Effects of Combined Testosterone and Finasteride Administration in Older Hypogonadal Men: A Randomized Controlled Trial," *Am J Physiol Endocrinol Metab*, February 2014.

13. K. Shigehara et al., "Effects of Testosterone Replacement Therapy on Hypogonadal Men with Osteopenia or Osteoporosis: A Subanalysis of

a Prospective Randomized Controlled Study in Japan," *Aging Male*, September 2017.

14. P. J. Snyder et al., "Effect of Testosterone Treatment on Volumetric Bone Density and Strength in Older Men with Low Testosterone: A Controlled Clinical Trial," *JAMA Intern Med*, April 2017.

Chapter Seven: Rebuilding Muscle Mass

1. M. Eichholzer et al., "Serum Sex Steroids Hormones and Frailty in Older American Men of the Third National Health and Nutrition Examination Survey," *Aging Male*, December 2012.

2. C. N. Roy et al., "Association of Testosterone Levels with Anemia in Older Men: A Controlled Clinical Trial," *JAMA Intern Med*, April 2017.

3. W. J. Karemer et al., "Hormonal Responses and Adaptations to Resistance Exercise and Training," *Sports Med*, 2005.

4. W. J. Kraemer et al., "Effects of Heavy-Resistance Training on Hormonal Response Patterns in Younger vs. Older Men," *J Appl Physiol*, September 1999.

5. E. Scudese et al., "Long Rest Interval Promotes Durable Testosterone Responses in High-Intensity Bench Press," *J Strength Cond Res*, May 2016.

6. D. A. Rubin et al., "Endocrine Response to Acute Resistance Exercise in Obese Versus Lean Physically Active Men," *Eur J Appl Physiol*, June 2015.

7. S. M. Ebert et al., "Identification and Small Molecule Inhibition of an Activating Transcription Factor 4 (ATF4)-Dependent Pathway to Age-Related Skeletal Muscle Weakness and Atrophy," *J Biol Chem*, October 2015.

8. "Keeping Older Muscles Strong," University of Iowa Health Care, September 8, 2015.

9. D. W. Frederick et al., "Loss of NAD Homeostasis Leads to Progressive and Reversible Degeneration of Skeletal Muscle," *Cell Metabolism*, August 2016.

10. K. L. Herbst et al., "Testosterone Action on Skeletal Muscle," *Curr Opin Clin Nutr Metab Care*, May 2004.

11. L. Frederiksen et al., "Testosterone Therapy Increased Muscle Mass and Lipid Oxidation in Aging Men," *Age*, February 2012.

12. T. W. Storer et al., "Effects of Testosterone Supplementation for 3 Years on Muscle Performance and Physical Function in Older Men," *J Clin Endorcinol Metab*, February 2017.

13. S. Bhasin et al., "Effect of Testosterone Replacement on Measures of Mobility in Older Men with Mobility Limitation and Low Testosterone

Concentrations: Secondary Analyses of the Testosterone Trials," *Lancet Diabetes Endrocinol*, November 2018.

14. J. W. Skinner et al., "Muscular Responses to Testosterone Replacement Vary by Administration Route: A Systematic Review and Meta-Analysis," *J Cachexia Sarcopenia Muscle*, June 2018.

Chapter Eight: Slowing Hair Thinning

1. "Androgenetic Alopecia," U.S. National Library of Medicine, https://ghr.nlm.nih,gov/condition/androgenetic-alopecia#genes (accessed 11/11/18).

2. "Testosterone, Prostate Cancer, and Balding: Is There a Link?" Harvard Health Publishing, January 23, 2017, https://www.health.harvard.edu/mens-health/testosterone-prostate-cancer-and-balding-is-there-a-link-thefamilyhealth-guide (accessed 11/11/18).

3. E. A. Olsen et al., "The Importance of Dual 5x-Reductase Inhibition in the Treatment of Male Pattern Hair Loss: Results of a Randomized Placebo-Controlled Study of Dutasteride versus Finasteride," *J Am Acad Dermaol*, December 2006.

4. H. W. Gudelin et al., "A Randomized, Active- and Placebo-Controlled Study of the Efficacy and Safety of Different Doses of Dutasteride versus Placebo and Finasteride in the Treatment of Male Subjects with Androgenetic Alopecia," *J Am Acad Dermaol*, March 2014.

5. V. L. Truong et al., "Hair Regenerative Mechanisms of Red Ginseng Oil and Its Major Components in the Testosterone-Induced Delay of Anagen Entry in C57BL/6 Mice," *Molecules*, September 2017.

6. B. Min-Ji et al., "Safety of Red Ginseng Oil for Single Oral Administration in Sprague-Dawley Rats," *J Ginseng Res*, January 2014.

7. J. L. Kang et al., "Promotion Effect of *Schisandra nigra* on the Growth of Hair," *Eur J Dermaol*, March–April 2009.

8. S. C. Kim, "Promotion Effect of Norgalanthamine, a Component of *Crinum asiaticum*, on Hair Growth," *Eur J Dermaol*, January–February 2010.

9. N. N. Zhang et al., "Hair Growth-Promoting Activity of Hot Water Extract of *Thuja orientalis*," *BMC Complement Altern Med*, January 2013.

10. K. Datta et al., "*Eclipta alba* Extract with Potential for Hair Growth Promoting Activity," *J Ethnoparmacol*, July 2009.

11. G. Brotzu et al., "A Liposome-Based Formulation Containing Equol, Dihomo-y-linolenic Acid (DGLA), and Propionyl-L-carnitine to Prevent and Treat Hair Loss: A Prospective Investigation," *Dermaol Ther*, October 2018.

Chapter Nine: Overcoming Fatigue

1. A. C. Hackney, "Effects of Endurance Exercise on the Reproductive System of Men: The 'Exercise-Hypogonadal Male Condition,'" *J Endocrinol Inv*, October 2008.

2. L. Di Luigi et al., "Prevalence of Undiagnosed Testosterone Deficiency in Aging Athletes: Does Exercise Training Influence the Symptoms of Male Hypogonadism?" *J Sex Med*, July 2010.

3. R. O. Van Heukelom et al., "Influence of Melatonin on Fatigue Severity in Patients with Chronic Fatigue Syndrome and Late Melatonin Secretion," *Eur J Neurology*, January 2006.

4. "Vitamin B12: Fact Sheet for Health Professionals," U.S. National Institutes of Health, Office of Dietary Supplements, https://ods.od.nih.gov/factsheets/VitaminB12-HealthProfessional/ (accessed 12/1/18).

5. R. Sainj, "Coenzyme Q10: The Essential Nutrient," *J Pharm Bioallied Sci*, July–September 2011.

6. S. K. Hung et al., "The Effectiveness and Efficacy of *Rhodiola rosea* L: A Systematic Review of Randomized Clinical Trials," *Phytomedicine*, February 2011.

7. M. A. Pratte et al., "An Alternative Treatment for Anxiety: A Systematic Review of Human Trial Results Reported for the Ayurvedic Herb Ashwagandha (*Withania somnifera*)," *J Altern Complement Med*, December 2014.

8. S. Shenoy et al., "Effects of Eight-Week Supplementation of Ashwagandha on Cardiorespiratory Endurance in Elite Indian Cyclists," *J Ayurveda Integr Med*, October 2012.

9. R. J. Maughan, "Impact of Mild Dehydration on Wellness and on Exercise Performance," *Eur J Clin Nutr*, December 2003.

10. C. Anderson and J. A. Horne, "A High Sugar Content, Low Caffeine Drink Does Not Alleviate Sleepiness but May Worsen It," *Hum Psychopharmacol*, July 2006.

11. E. Del Fabbro et al., "Testosterone Replacement for Fatigue in Hypgonadal Ambulatory Males with Advanced Cancer: A Preliminary Double-Blind Placebo-Controlled Trial," *Support Care Cancer*, September 2013.

12. R. M. Bercea et al., "Fatigue and Serum Testosterone in Obstructive Sleep Apnea Patients," *Clin Respir J*, July 2015.

13. U. S. Shankar et al., "Effects of Testosterone on Muscle Strength, Physical Function, Body Composition, and Quality of Life in Intermediate-Frail and Frail Elderly Men: A Randomized, Double-Blind, Placebo-Controlled Study," *J of Clin Endocrin Metabolism*, February 2010.

Chapter Ten: Managing Chronic Stress

1. K. Hirokawa et al., "Job Demands as a Potential Modifier of the Association between Testosterone Deficiency and Andropause Symptoms in Japanese Middle-Aged Workers: A Cross-Sectional Study," *Maturitas*, November 2012.

2. K. Hirokawa et al., "Modification Effects of Changes in Job Demands on Associations between Changes in Testosterone Levels and Andropause Symptoms: 2-Year Follow-up Study in Male Middle-Aged Japanese Workers," *Int J Behav Med*, August 2016.

3. E. Tachikawa and K. Kudo, "Proof of the Mysterious Efficacy of Ginseng: Basic and Clinical Trials: Suppression of Adrenal Medullary Function in Vitro by Ginseng," *J Pharmacol Sci*, June 2004.

4. T. E. Palisin and J. J. Stacy, "Ginseng: Is It in the Root?" *Curr Sports Med Rep*, June 2006.

5. K. T. Choi, "Botanical Characteristics, Pharmacological Effects and Medicinal Components of Korean Panax Ginseng CA Meyer," *Acta Parmacol Sin*, September 2008.

6. B. Kocaadam et al., "Curcumin, an Active Component of Turmeric (*Curcuma longa*), and Its Effects on Health," *Crit Rev Food Sci Nutr*, 2017.

7. A. Wu et al., "Curcumin Boosts DHA in the Brain: Implications for the Prevention of Anxiety Disorders," *Biochim Biophys Acta*, May 2015.

8. S. H. Kim et al., "Laughter and Stress Relief in Cancer Patients: A Pilot Study," *Evid Based Complent Alt Med*, 2015.

9. Y. Fujiwara et al., "Hearing Laughter Improves the Recovery Process of the Autonomic Nervous System after a Stress-Loading Task: A Randomized Controlled Trial," *Biopsychosoc Med*, December 2018.

10. L. Lin et al., "The Effects of a Modified Mindfulness-Based Stress Reduction Program for Nurses: A Randomized Controlled Trial," *Workplace Health*, October 2018.

11. S. F. Nery et al., "Mindfulness-Based Program for Stress Reduction in Infertile Women: Randomized Controlled Trial," *Stress Health*, October 2018.

12. M. C. Pascoe et al., "Yoga, Mindfulness-Based Stress Reduction and Stress-Related Physiological Measures: A Meta-analysis," *Psychoneuroendocrinology*, December 2017.

Chapter Eleven: Countering Sleep Decline

1. A. J. Clark et al., "Onset of Impaired Sleep as a Predictor of Change in Health-Related Behaviours: Analyzing Observational Data as a Series of Non-Randomized Pseudo-Trials," *Int J Epidemiol*, June 2015.

2. R. Luboshitzky et al., "Disruption of the Nocturnal Testosterone Rhythm by Sleep Fragmentation in Normal Men," *J Clin Endocrinol Metab*, March 2001.

3. Luboshitzky et al., "Disruption of the Nocturnal Testosterone Rhythm."

4. O. Burschtin and J. Wang, "Testosterone Deficiency and Sleep Apnea," *Sleep Med Clin*, December 2016.

5. S. D. Kim and K. S. Cho, "Obstructive Sleep Apnea and Testosterone Deficiency," *World J Men's Health*, January 2019.

6. I. M. Madaeva et al., "Obstructive Sleep Apnea Syndrome and Age-Related Hypogonadism," *Zh Nevrol Psikhiatra Im S Korsakova*, 2017.

7. Z. Xie et al., "A Review of Sleep Disorders and Melatonin," *Neurol Res*, June 2017.

8. W. Shell et al., "A Randomized Placebo-Controlled Trial of an Amino Acid Preparation on Timing and Quality of Sleep," *Am J Therapeutics*, March–April 2010.

9. G. Howatson et al., "Effect of Tart Cherry Juice (*Prunus cerasus*) on Melatonin Levels and Enhanced Sleep Quality," *European Journal of Nutrition*, December 2012.

10. H. Cao et al., "Acupuncture for Treatment of Insomnia: A Systematic Review of Randomized Controlled Trials," *J Alt Comple Med*, 2009.

11. M. L. Chen et al., "The Effectiveness of Acupressure in Improving the Quality of Sleep of Institutionalized Residents," *J Gerontology Biol Sci*, 1999.

12. A. Bowden et al., "Autogenic Training as a Behavioural Approach to Insomnia: A Prospective Study," *Primary Health Care Research & Development*, April 2012.

13. "Cognitive Behavioral Therapy for Insomnia," National Sleep Foundation, https://www.sleepfoundation.org/sleep-news/cognitive-behavioral -therapy-insomnia (accessed 1/4/19).

14. J. W. Trauer et al., "Cognitive Behavioral Therapy for Chronic Insomnia: A Systematic Review and Meta-Analysis," *Annals Internal Medicine*, 2015.

15. A. G. Harvey and S. Payne, "The Management of Unwanted Presleep Thoughts in Insomnia: Distraction with Imagery versus General Distraction," *Behav Res Ther*, March 2002.

16. D. S. Black et al., "Mindfulness Meditation and Improvement in Sleep Quality and Daytime Impairment Among Older Adults with Sleep Disturbances: A Randomized Clinical Trial," *JAMA Intern Med*, 2015.

17. "Sleep, Stress and Relaxation," University of California, Davis, https://shcs.ucdavis.edu/sites/default/files/documents/conquering_insomnia_session -04.pdf (accessed 1/8/19).

18. G. D. Jacobs, "Clinical Applications of the Relaxation Response and Mind-Body Interventions," *J Altern Complement Med*, 2001.

19. C. E. Milner and K. Cote, "Benefits of Napping in Healthy Adults: Impact of Nap Length, Time of Day, Age, and Experience with Napping," *Journal of Sleep Research*, May 2009.

Chapter Twelve: Stopping Breast Growth

1. R. E. Johnson and H. Murad, "Gynecomastia: Pathophysiology, Evaluation, and Management," *Mayo Clin Proc*, November 2009.

2. S. L. Hines et al., "The Role of Mammography in Male Patients with Breast Symptoms," *Mayo Clin Proc*, 2007.

3. V. Purohit, "Can Alcohol Promote Aromatization of Androgens to Estrogens? A Review," *Alcohol*, November 2000.

4. K. Watanabe et al., "Marijuana Extracts Possess the Effects Like the Endocrine Disrupting Chemicals," *Toxicology*, January 2005.

5. S. A. Brody and D. L. Loriaux, "Epidemic of Gynecomastia among Haitian Refugees: Exposure to an Environmental Antiandrogen," *Endocr Pract*, September 2003.

6. J. Martinez and J. E. Lewi, "An Unusual Case of Gynecomastia Associated with Soy Product Consumption," *Endocr Pract*, May–June 2008.

7. "Enlarged Breasts in Men (Gynecomastia): Overview," Mayo Clinic, https://www.mayoclinic.org (accessed 1/12/19).

8. A. Dobs and M. J. Darkes, "Incidence and Management of Gynecomastia in Men Treated for Prostate Cancer," *J Urol*, November 2005.

9. G. S. Mannu et al., "Role of Tamoxifen in Idiopathic Gynecomastia: A 10-Year Prospective Cohort Study," *Breast J*, November 2018.

10. E. H. Courtiss, "Gynecomastia: Analysis of 159 Patients and Current Recommendations for Treatment," *Plast Reconstr Surg*, May 1987.

11. A. C. Prado and P. F. Castillo, "Minimal Surgical Access to Treat Gynecomastia with the Use of a Power-Assisted Arthroscopic-Endoscopic Cartilage Shaver," *Plast Reconstr Surg*, March 2005.

Chapter Thirteen: Reversing Weight Gain

1. A. Haider et al., "Hypogonadal Obese Men with and without Diabetes Mellitus Type 2 Lose Weight and Show Improvement in Cardiovascular Risk Factors When Treated with Testosterone: An Observational Study," *Obes Res Clin Pract*, July–August 2014.

2. E. M. Carmacho, "Age-Associated Changes in Hypothalamic-Pituitary-Testicular Function in Middle-Aged and Older Men Are Modified by Weight

Change and Lifestyle Factors: Longitudinal Results from the European Male Ageing Study," *Eur J Endocrinol*, February 2013.

3. L. Antonio et al., "Associations between Sex Steroids and the Development of Metabolic Syndrome: A Longitudinal Study in European Men," *J Clin Endocrinol Metab*, April 2015.

4. R. Kelishadi et al., "Role of Environmental Chemicals in Obesity: A Systematic Review on the Current Evidence," *J Environ Public Health*, 2013.

5. M. Ezzati et al., "Trends in Adult Body-Mass Index in 200 Countries from 1975 to 2014: A Pooled Analysis of 1698 Population-Based Measurement Studies with 19.2 Million Participants," *The Lancet*, April 2016.

6. J. J. Heindel et al., "Endocrine Disruptors and Obesity," *Nat Rev. Endocrinol*, November 2015.

7. O. Yang et al., "Endocrine-Disrupting Chemicals: Review of Toxicological Mechanisms Using Molecular Pathway Analysis," *J Cancer Prev*, March 2015.

8. S. J. Genuis et al., "Human Excretion of Bisphenol A: Blood, Urine, Sweat Study," *J Environ Public Health*, 2012.

9. "Types of Bariatric Surgery," National Institute of Diabetes and Digestive and Kidney Diseases, https://www.niddk.nih.gov/health-information/weight-management/bariatric-surgery/types (accessed 1/14/19).

10. A. P. Courcoulas et al., "Weight Change and Health Outcomes at 3 Years after Bariatric Surgery among Individuals with Severe Obesity," *Journal of the American Medical Association*, 2013.

11. G. Corona et al., "Body Weight Loss Reverts Obesity-Associated Hypogonadotropic Hypogonadism: A Systematic Review and Meta-analysis," *Eur J Endocrinol*, May 2013.

12. G. Corona et al., "Testosterone Supplementation and Body Composition: Results from a Meta-analysis Study," *European Society of Endocrinology*, November 2015.

13. E. B. Schmitt et al., "Vitamin D Deficiency Is Associated with Metabolic Syndrome in Postmenopausal Women," *Maturitas*, January 2018.

14. R. Rafiq et al., "Associations of Different Body Fat Deposits with Serum 25-Hydroxyvitamin D Concentrations," *European Society of Endocrinology*, 2018.

15. D. T. Dibaba et al., "Dietary Magnesium Intake and Risk of Metabolic Syndrome: A Meta-analysis," *Diabet Med*, November 2014.

16. R. De la Iglesia et al., "Dietary Strategies Implicated in the Prevention and Treatment of Metabolic Syndrome," *Int J Mol Sci*, November 2016.

17. L. J. Moran et al., "Long-Term Effects of a Randomised Controlled Trial Comparing High Protein or High Carbohydrate Weight Loss Diets

on Testosterone, SHBG, Erectile and Urinary Function in Overweight and Obese Men," *PLOS One*, September 2016.

18. D. M. Schulte et al., "Caloric Restriction Increases Serum Testosterone Concentrations in Obese Male Subjects by Two Distinct Mechanisms," *Horm Metab Res*, 2014.

19. De la Iglesia et al., "Dietary Strategies Implicated."

20. S. G. Lee et al., "Panax Ginseng Leaf Extracts Exert Anti-Obesity Effects in High-Fat Diet-Induced Obese Rats," *Nutrients*, September 2017.

21. S. S. Shin and M. Yoon, "Korean Red Ginseng (Panax Ginseng) Inhibits Obesity and Improves Lipid Metabolism in High Fat Diet-Fed Castrated Mice," *J Ethnopharmacol*, January 2018.

22. F. Saad et al., "Effects of Long-Term Treatment with Testosterone on Weight and Waist Size in 411 Hypogonadal Men with Obesity Classes 1-III: Observational Data from Two Registry Studies," *Int J Obes*, January 2016.

23. F. Saad et al., "Testosterone as Potential Effective Therapy in Treatment of Obesity in Men with Testosterone Deficiency: A Review," *Curr Diabetes Rev*, March 2012.

24. A. M. Traish, "Testosterone and Weight Loss: The Evidence," *Curr Opin Endocrinol Diabetes Obes*, October 2014.

25. A. M. Traish et al., "Long-Term Testosterone Therapy in Hypogonadal Men Ameliorates Elements of the Metabolic Syndrome: An Observational, Long-Term Registry Study," *Int J Clin Pract*, March 2014.

Chapter Fourteen: Treating Prostate Problems

1. "Benign Prostatic Hyperplasia: Overview," Mayo Clinic, https://www.mayoclinic.org/diseases-conditions/benign-prostatic-hyperplasia/symptoms-causes/syc-20370087 (accessed 1/18/19).

2. "Prostatitis: Overview," Mayo Clinic, https://www.mayoclinic.org/diseases-conditions/prostatitis/symptoms-causes/syc-20355766 (accessed 1/19/19).

3. D. Cui et al., "The Effect of Chronic Prostatitis on Zinc Concentration of Prostatic Fluid and Seminal Plasma: A Systematic Review and Meta-analysis," *Curr Med Res Opin*, 2015.

4. D. Tiscione et al., "Daidzein Plus Isolase Associated with Zinc Improves Clinical Symptoms and Quality of Life in Patients with LUTS Due to benign Prostatic Hyperplasia: Results from a Phase 1-II Study," *Arch Ital Urol Androl*, March 2017.

5. A. Fallah et al., "Zinc Is an Essential Element for Male Fertility: A Review of Zn Roles in Men's Health, Germination, Sperm Quality, and Fertilization," *J Reprod Infertil*, April–June 2018.

6. L. R. Brilla et al., "Effects of a Novel Zinc-Magnesium Formulation on Hormones and Strength," *J Exercise Phys*, October 2000.

7. K. Koehler et al., "Serum Testosterone and Urinary Excretion of Steroid Hormone Metabolites after Administration of a High Dose Zinc Supplement," *Eur J Clin Nutr*, 2009.

8. A. Gonzalez et al., "Zinc Intake from Supplements and Diet and Prostate Cancer," *Nutr Cancer*, 2009.

9. A. M. Mahmoud et al., "Zinc Intake and Risk of Prostate Cancer: Case-Control Study and Meta-Analysis," *PLOS One*, November 2016.

10. P. Christudoss et al., "Zinc Status of Patients with Benign Prostatic Hyperplasia and Prostate Carcinoma," *Indian J Urol*, January–March 2011.

11. M. R. Safarineiad, "Urtica Dioica for Treatment of Benign Prostatic Hyperplasia: A Prospective, Randomized, Double-Blind, Placebo-Controlled, Crossover Study," *J Herb Pharmacother*, 2005.

12. A. Nahata et al., "Ameliorative Effects of Stinging Nettle (*Urtica dioica*) on Testosterone-Induced Prostatic Hyperplasia in Rats," *Andrologia*, May 2012.

13. L. S. Marks et al., "Effects of a Saw Palmetto Herbal Blend in Men with Symptomatic Benign Prostatic Hyperplasia," *J Urol*, May 2000.

14. H. G. Preuss et al., "Randomized Trial of a Combination of Natural Products (Cernitin, Saw Palmetto, B-Sitosterol, Vitamin E) on Symptoms of Benign Prostatic Hyperplasia (BPH)," *Int Urol Nephrol*, 2001.

15. J. Tacklind et al., "*Serenoa repens* for Benign Prostatic Hyperplasia," *Cochrane Database Syst Rev*, December 2012.

16. A. Russo et al., "*Sereno repens*, Selenium and Lycopene to Manage Lower Urinary Tract Symptoms Suggestive for Benign Prostatic Hyperplasia," *Expert Opin Drug Saf*, December 2016.

17. S. L. Ooi and S. C. Pak, "*Serenoa repens* for Lower Urinary Tract Symptoms/Benign Prostatic Hyperplasia: Current Evidence and Its Clinical Implications in Naturopathic Medicine," *J Altern Complement Med*, August 2017.

18. W. Vahlensieck et al., "Effects of Pumpkin Seed in Men with Lower Urinary Tract Symptoms Due to Benign Prostatic Hyperplasia in the One-Year, Randomized, Placebo-Controlled GRANU Study," *Urol Int*, 2015.

19. R. Damiano et al., "The Role of Cucurbita Pepo in the Management of Patients Affected by Lower Urinary Tract Symptoms Due to Benign Prostatic Hyperplasia: A Narrative Review," *Arch Ital Urol Androl*, July 2016.

20. T. J. Walsh et al., "Testosterone Treatment and the Risk of Aggressive Prostate Cancer in Men with Low Testosterone Levels," *PLOS One*, June 2018.

21. F. M. Debruyne et al., "Testosterone Treatment Is Not Associated with Increased Risk of Prostate Cancer or Worsening of Lower Urinary Tract Symptoms: Prostate Health Outcomes in the Registry of Hypogonadism in Men," *BJC Int*, February 2017.

22. V. Golla and A. L. Kaplan, "Testosterone Therapy on Active Surveillance and Following Definitive Treatment for Prostate Cancer," *Curr Urol Rep*, July 2017.

23. W. Baas and T. S. Kohler, "Testosterone Replacement Therapy and BPH/LUTS. What Is the Evidence?" *Curr Urol Rep*, June 2016.

24. K. J. DeLay and T. S. Kohler, "Testosterone and the Prostate: Artifacts and Truths," *Urol Clin North Am*, August 2016.

Chapter Fifteen: Restoring Male Sexual Function

1. Y. Luo et al., "Sex Hormones Predict the Incidence of Erectile Dysfunction: From a Population-Based Prospective Cohort Study (FAMHES)," *J Sex Med*, May 2015.

2. M. Schulster et al., "The Role of Estradiol in Male Reproductive Function," *Asian J Androl*, May–June 2016.

3. J. S. Finkelstein et al., "Gonadal Steroids and Body Composition, Strength, and Sexual Function in Men," *New Eng J Med*, September 2013.

4. M. L. Anderson et al., "The Association of Testosterone, Sleep, and Sexual Function in Men and Women," *Brain Research*, October 2011.

5. A. M. Traish et al., "The Dark Side of Testosterone Deficiency: Metabolic Syndrome and Erectile Dysfunction," *J Androl*, January–February 2009.

6. G. Jackson et al., "The Assessment of Vascular Risk in Men with Erectile Dysfunction: The Role of the Cardiologist and General Physician," *Int J Clin Pract*, November 2013.

7. J. Basu and S. Sharma, "Erectile Dysfunction Heralds Onset of Cardiovascular Disease," *Practitioner*, June 2016.

8. I. Gruenwald et al., "Shockwave Treatment of Erectile Dysfunction," *Ther Adv Urol*, April 2013.

9. J. Khoo et al., "Comparing Effects of Low- and High-Volume Moderate-Intensity Exercise on Sexual Function and Testosterone in Obese Men," *J Sex Med*, July 2013.

10. A. B. Silva et al., "Physical Activity and Exercise for Erectile Dysfunction: Systematic Review and Meta-analysis," *Br J Sports Med*, October 2017.

11. F. Giugliano et al., "Adherence to Mediterranean Diet and Erectile Dysfunction in Men with Type 2 Diabetes," *J Sex Med*, May 2010.

12. K. Esposito et al., "Dietary Factors, Mediterranean Diet and Erectile Dysfunction," *J Sex Med*, July 2010.

13. P. A. Della Camera et al., "Sexual Health, Adherence to Mediterranean Diet, Body Weight, Physical Activity and Mental State: Factors Correlated to Each Other," *Urologia*, October 2017.

14. F. Wang et al., "Erectile Dysfunction and Fruit/Vegetable Consumption among Diabetic Canadian Men," *Urology*, December 2013.

15. O. Canguven et al., "Vitamin D Treatment Improves Levels of Sexual Hormones, Metabolic Parameters and Erectile Function in Middle-Aged Vitamin D Deficient Men," *Aging Male*, March 2017.

16. G. Tirabassi et al., "Vitamin D and Male Sexual Function: A Transversal and Longitudinal Study," *Int J Endocrinol*, January 2018.

17. E. Lerchbaum et al., "Effects of Vitamin D Supplementation on Androgens in Men with Low Testosterone Levels: A Randomized Controlled Trial," *Eur J Nutr*, November 2018.

18. G. F. Gonzales et al., "Effect of *Lepidium meyenii* (Maca), a Root with Aphrodisiac and Fertility-Enhancing Properties, on Serum Reproductive Hormone Levels in Adult Healthy Men," *J Endocrinol*, January 2003.

19. S. Beharry and M. J. Heinrich, "Is the Hype around the Reproductive Health Claims of Maca (*Lepidium meyenil* Walp.) Justified?" *Ethnopharmacol*, January 2018.

20. V. Neychev and V. Mitev, "Pro-sexual and Androgen Enhancing Effects of *Tribulus terrestris* L.: Fact or Fiction," *J Ethnaopharmacol*, February 2016.

21. W. Zhu et al., "A Review of Traditional Pharmacological Uses, Phytochemistry, and Pharmacological Activities of *Tribulus terrestris*," *Chem Cent J*, 2017.

22. S. Hirsh et al., "An Open Label Study to Evaluate the Effect of *Kaempferia parviflora* in Support of Erectile Function and Male Sexual Health among Overall Healthy Males 50–70," *FASEB J*, April 2017.

23. R. A. Stei et al., "*Kaempferia parviflora* Ethanol Extract Improves Self-Assessed Sexual Health in Men: A Pilot Study," *J Int Med*, July 2018.

24. M. Tambi et al., "Standardised Water-Soluble Extract of *Eurycoma longifolia*, as Testosterone Booster for Managing Men with Late-Onset Hypogonadism?" *Andrologia*, May 2012.

25. A. George and R. Henkel, "Phytoandrogenic Properties of *Eurycoma longifolia* as Natural Alternative to Testosterone Replacement Therapy," *Andrologia*, September 2014.

26. S. Kotirum et al., "Efficacy of Tongkat Ali (*Eurycoma longifolia*) on Erectile Function Improvement: Systematic Review and Meta-analysis of Randomized Controlled Trials," *Complement Ther Med*, October 2015.

27. B. Hong et al., "A Double-Blind Crossover Study Evaluating the Efficacy of Korean Red Ginseng in Patients with Erectile Dysfunction: A Preliminary Report," *J Urol*, November 2002.

28. E. De Andrade et al., "Study of the Efficacy of Korean Red Ginseng in the Treatment of Erectile Dysfunction," *Asian J Androl*, March 2007.

29. D. J. Jang et al., "Red Ginseng for Treating Erectile Dysfunction: A Systematic Review," *Br J Clin Pharmacol*, October 2008.

30. Y. D. Choi et al., "Effects of Korean Ginseng Berry Extract on Sexual Function in Men with Erectile Dysfunction: A Multicenter, Placebo-Controlled, Double-Blind Clinical Study," *Int J Impot Res*, March–April 2013.

31. E. Steels et al., "Physiological Aspects of Male Libido Enhanced by Standardized *Trigonella foenum-graecum* Extract and Mineral Formulation," *Phytother Res*, September 2011.

32. A. Rao et al., "Testofen, a Specialized *Trigonella foenum-graecum* Seed Extract Reduces Age-Related Symptoms of Androgen Decrease, Increases Testosterone Levels and Improves Sexual Function in Healthy Aging Males in a Double-Blind Randomized Clinical Study," *Aging Male*, June 2016.

33. A. Maheshwari et al., "Efficacy of Furosap™, a Novel *Trigonella foenum-graecum* Seed Extract, in Enhancing Testosterone Level and Improving Sperm Profile in Male Volunteers," *Int J Med Sci*, January 2017.

34. W. J. Bae et al., "Antioxidant and Antifibrotic Effect of a Herbal Formulation in Vitro and in the Experimental Andropause via Nrf2/HO-1 Signaling Pathway," *Oxid Med Cell Longev*, 2017.

35. K. W. Lee et al., "A Randomized, Controlled Study of Treatment with Ojayeonjonghwan for Patients with Late Onset Hypogonadism," *Aging Male*, July 2018.

36. S. W. Choi et al., "Effect of Korean Herbal Formula (Modified Ojayeonjonghwan) on Androgen Receptor Expression in an Aging Rat Model of Late Onset Hypogonadism," *World J Men's Health*, January 2019.

37. G. R. Shah et al., "Evaluation of a Multi-herb Supplement for Erectile Dysfunction: A Randomized Double-Blind, Placebo-Controlled Study," *BMC Complement Altern Med*, September 2012.

38. M. Khera et al., "Improved Sexual Function with Testosterone Replacement Therapy in Hypogonadal Men: Real-World Data from the Testim Registry in the United States," *J Sex Med,* November 2011.

39. D. J. Yassin et al., "Long-Term Testosterone Treatment in Elderly Men with Hypogonadism and Erectile Dysfunction Reduces Obesity Parameters and Improves Metabolic Syndrome and Health-Related Quality of Life," *J Sex Med*, June 2014.

40. G. R. Cunningham et al., "Association of Sex Hormones with Sexual Function, Vitality, and Physical Function of Symptomatic Older Men with Low Testosterone Levels at Baseline in the Testosterone Trials," *J Clin Endocrinol Metab*, March 2015.

41. G. R. Cunningham et al., "Testosterone Treatment and Sexual Function in Older Men with Low Testosterone Levels," *J Clin Endocrinol Metab*, August 2016.

42. G. Corona et al., "Meta-analysis of Results of Testosterone Therapy on Sexual Function Based on International Index of Erectile Function Scores," *Eur Urol*, December 2017.

Chapter Sixteen: About Testosterone Replacement Therapy

1. M. Balliett and J. R. Burke, "Changes in Anthropometric Measurements, Body Composition, Blood Pressure, Lipid Profile, and Testosterone in Patients Participating in a Low-Energy Dietary Intervention," *J Chirop Med*, March 2013.

2. Y. Oi et al., "Garlic Supplementation Increases Testicular Testosterone and Decreases Plasma Corticosterone in Rats Fed a High Protein Diet," *J Nutr*, August 2001.

3. K. K. Shukla et al., "*Mucuna pruriens* Improves Male Fertility by Its Actions on the Hypothalamus-Pituitary-Gonadal Axis," *Fertil Steril*, December 2009.

4. S. Pandit et al., "Clinical Evaluation of Purified Shilajit on Testosterone Levels in Healthy Volunteers," *Andrologia*, January 2016.

5. N. Samaras et al., "Off-Label Use of Hormones as an Anti-aging Strategy: A Review," *Clinical Interventions in Aging*, 2014.

6. Kenneth Janson, "Benefits of Hormone Replacement Therapy," PrevientMD, www.myhealthengage.com, 2016 (accessed 1/31/19).

7. R. Heidari et al., "Can Testosterone Level Be a Good Predictor of Late-Onset Hypogonadism?" *Andrologia*, May 2015.

8. I. T. Huhtaniemi, "Andropause—Lessons from the European Male Ageing Study," *Annals of Endocrinology*, May 2014.

9. K. B. Luthy and C. Williams, "Comparison of Testosterone Replacement Therapy Medications for Treatment of Hypogonadism," *J Nurse Pract*, 2017.

10. J. J. Shoskesq et al., "Pharmacology and Testosterone Replacement Therapy Preparations," *Transl Androl Urol*, 2016 December.

11. A. Z. Vinarov et al., "Effect of Transdermal Testosterone on the Quality of Life of Men with Androgen Deficiency and Chronic Prostatitis in Routine Clinical Practice," *Urologia*, March 2018.

12. T. McNicholas and T. Ong, "Review of Testim Gel," *Expert Opin Pharmacother*, March 2016.

13. L. Belkoff et al., "Efficacy and Safety of Testosterone Replacement Gel for Treating Hypogonadism in Men: Phase III Open-Label Studies," *Andrologia*, February 2018.

14. M. Carruthers et al., "Evolution of Testosterone Treatment over 25 Years: Symptom Responses, Endocrine Profiles and Cardiovascular Changes," *Aging Male*, 2015.

15. "Bioidentical Hormones," Cleveland Clinic, www.clevelandclinic.org/health/articles/15660-bioidentical-hormones (accessed 1/22/19).

16. K. Holtorf, "The Bioidentical Hormone Debate: Are Bioidentical Hormones (Estradiol, Estriol, And Progesterone) Safer or More Efficacious Than Commonly Used Synthetic Versions in Hormone Replacement Therapy?" *Postgard Med*, January 2009.

17. "Bioidentical Hormones: Are They Safer?" Mayo Clinic, https://www.mayoclinic.org/diseases-conditions/menopause/expert-answers/bioidentical-hormones/faq-20058460 (accessed 1/22/19).

18. Paul Ling Tai, "For a Younger Tomorrow: Saliva Hormone Testing Is The First Step to Extending Your Youthful Years," *Healing Our World* 38, no. 4, October 2018, www.hippocratesinstituate.org.

19. M. L. Eisenberg, "Testosterone Replacement Therapy and Prostate Cancer Incidence," *World J Men's Health*, December 2015.

20. J. Klap et al., "The Relationship between Total Testosterone Levels and Prostate Cancer: A Review of the Continuing Controversy," *J Urol*, February 2015.

21. Y. Cui and Y. Zhang, "The Effect of Androgen-Replacement Therapy On Prostate Growth: A Systematic Review and Meta-analysis," *Eur Urol*, November 2013.

22. F. M. Debruyne et al., "Testosterone Treatment Is Not Associated with Increased Risk of Prostate Cancer or Worsening of Lower Urinary Tract Symptoms: Prostate Health Outcomes in the Registry of Hypogonadism in Men," *BJU Int*, February 2017.

23. S. Loeb et al., "Testosterone Replacement Therapy and Risk of Favorable and Aggressive Prostate Cancer," *J Clin Oncol*, May 2017.

24. "Testosterone Therapy Does Not Raise Risk of Aggressive Prostate Cancer," *ScienceDaily*, May 7, 2016, www.sciencedaily.com/releases/2016/05/160507143326.htm (3/15/2019).

25. A. M. Traish et al., "The Dark Side of Testosterone Deficiency: III. Cardiovascular Disease," *J Androl*, September–October 2009.

26. T. C. Cheetham et al., "Association of Testosterone Replacement with Cardiovascular Outcomes among Men with Androgen Deficiency," *JAMA Intern Med*, April 2017.

27. A, M, Traish et al., "Long-Term Testosterone Therapy Improves Cardiometabolic Function and Reduces Risk of Cardiovascular Disease in Men with Hypogonadism: A Real-Life Observational Registry Study Setting Comparing Treated and Untreated (Control) Groups," *J Cardiovasc Pharmacol Ther*, September 2017.

28. T. H. Jones and D. M. Kelly, "Randomized Controlled Trials— Mechanistic Studies of Testosterone and the Cardiovascular System," *Asian J Androl*, March–April 2018.

29. A. Morgentaler, "Testosterone, Cardiovascular Risk, and Hormonophobia," *J Sex Med*, 2014.

30. R. Sharma et al., "Normalization of Testosterone Level Is Associated with Reduced Incidence of Myocardial Infarction and Mortality in Men," *European Heart Journal*, October 2015.

31. Sharma et al., "Normalization of Testosterone Level Is Associated with Reduced Incidence."

32. M. Toma et al., "Testosterone Supplementation in Heart Failure: A Meta-analysis," *Circ Heart Fail*, May 2012.

33. Sharma et al., "Normalization of Testosterone Level Is Associated with Reduced Incidence."

34. R. Sharma et al., "Normalization of Testosterone Levels after Testosterone Replacement Therapy Is Associated with Decreased Incidence of Atrial Fibrillation," *J Am Heart Association*, May 2017.

35. J. A. Pearl et al., "Testosterone Supplementation Does Not Worsen Urinary Tract Symptoms," *J Urol*, November 2013.

36. K. Okada et al., "Improved Lower Urinary Tract Symptoms Associated with Testosterone Replacement Therapy in Japanese Men with Late-Onset Hypogonadism," *Am J Men's Health*, June 2016.

37. T. P. Kohn et al., "Effects of Testosterone Replacement Therapy on Lower Urinary Tract Symptoms: A Systematic Review and Meta-analysis," *Eur Urol*, June 2016.

38. Kenneth Janson, "Decreasing the Risk of Cognitive Decline," *PrevientMD*, http://myhealthengage.com/blogs/view/220/decreasing-the-risk-of-cognitive-decline (accessed 1/25/19).

39. M. Maggio et al., "The Hormonal Pathway to Cognitive Impairment in Older Men," *Journal of Nutrition, Health and Aging*, 2012.

40. L. D. Baker et al., "Effects of Growth Hormone-Releasing Hormone on Cognitive Function in Adults with Mild Cognitive Impairment and Healthy Older Adults: Results of a Controlled Trial," *Archives of Neurology*, November 2012.

41. J. M. Daniel et al., "The Critical Period Hypothesis of Estrogen Effect On Cognition: Insights from Basic Research," *Biochimica et Biphysica Acta*, 2010.

42. G. Nave et al., "Single-Dose Testosterone Administration Impairs Cognitive Reflection in Men," *Psychological Science*, October 2017.

43. G. Nave et al., "Single-Dose Testosterone Administration Increases Men's Preference for Status Goods," *Nature Communications*, 2018.

44. W. Wang et al., "Cigarette Smoking Has a Positive and Independent Effect on Testosterone Levels," *Hormones*, October–December 2013.

45. A. Morales et al., "Androgens and Sexual Function: A Placebo-Controlled, Randomized, Double-Blind Study of Testosterone vs. Dehydroepiandrosterone in Men with Sexual Dysfunction and Androgen Deficiency," *Aging Male*, December 2009.

46. V. Martina et al., "Short-Term Dehydroepiandrosterone Treatment Increases Platelet cGMP Production in Elderly Male Subjects," *Clin Endocrinol (Oxf)*, March 2006.

47. M. B. Wallace et al., "Effects of Dehydroepiandrosterone vs. Androstenedione Supplementation in Men," *Med Sci Sports Exerc*, December 1999.

48. T. C. Liu et al., "Effect of Acute DHEA Administration on Free Testosterone in Middle-Aged and Young Men Following High-Intensity Interval Training," *Eur J Appl Physiol*, July 2013.

49. "The Best Testosterone Booster," Reviews.com, January 4, 2019, www.reviews.com/testosterone-booster/ (accessed 1/30/19).

50. J. R. Kovac et al., "Dietary Adjuncts for Improving Testosterone Levels in Hypogonadal Males," *Am J Men's Health*, August 2015.

51. R. Glaser and C. Dimitrakakis, "Testosterone Therapy in Women: Myths and Misconceptions," *Maturitas*, 2013.

52. M. Khera, "Testosterone Therapy for Female Sexual Dysfunction," *Sex Med Rev*, 2015.

53. C. Achilli et al., "Efficacy and Safety of Transdermal Testosterone in Postmenopausal Women with Hypoactive Sexual Desire Disorder: A Systematic Review and Meta-analysis," *Fertil Steril*, February 2017.

54. M. Gouveia et al., "The Role of Testosterone in the Improvement of Sexual Desire in Postmenopausal Women: An Evidence-Based Clinical Review," *Acta Med Port*, November 2018.

Chapter Seventeen: Can Human Growth Hormone Be Safely Replaced?

1. A. A. Toogood et al., "Beyond the Somatopause: Growth Hormone Deficiency in Adults Over the Age of 60 Years," *J Clin Endocrinol Met*, 1995.

2. A. Takeda et al., "Recombinant Human Growth Hormone for the Treatment of Growth Disorders in Children: A Systematic Review and Economic Evaluation," *Health Technol Assess*, September 2010.

3. "Off-Label Drug Use: What You Need to Know," WebMD, https://www.webmd.com/a-to-z-guides/features/off-label-drug-use-what-you-need-to-know#1 (accessed 2/1/19).

4. I. Mulligan et al., "Growth Hormone Doping: A Review," *Open Access J Sports Med*, July 2011.

5. G. P. Baumann GP, "Growth Hormone Doping in Sports: A Critical Review of Use and Detection Strategies," *Endocr Rev*, April 2012.

6. L. Zhanzhan et al., "Growth Hormone Replacement Therapy Reduces Risk of Cancer in Adult with Growth Hormone Deficiency: A Meta-analysis," *Oncotarget*, December 2016.

7. Derek Bagley, "Growing Concerns: A Look at Growth Hormone Research," *Endocrine News*, July 2016.

8. M. Barake et al., "Effects of Recombinant Human Growth Hormone Therapy on Bone Mineral Density in Adults with Growth Hormone Deficiency: A Meta-analysis," *J Clin Endocrinol Metab*, March 2014.

9. K. C. Mekala and N. A. Tritos, "Effects of Recombinant Human Growth Hormone Therapy in Obesity in Adults: A Meta Analysis," *J Clin Endocrinol Metab*, January 2009.

10. A. B. W. Tavares et al., "Effects of Growth Hormone Administration on Muscle Strength in Men over 50 Years Old," *Int J Endocrinol*, November 2013.

11. V. Z. Ajdzanovic et al., "Somatopause, Weaknesses of the Therapeutic Approaches and the Cautious Optimism Based on Experimental Ageing Studies with Soy Isoflavones," *EXCLI Journal*, March 2018.

12. M. L. Hartman et al., "Augmented Growth Hormone (GH) Secretory Burst Frequency and Amplitude Mediate Enhanced GH Secretion during a Two-Day Fast in Normal Men," *J Clin Endocrinol Met*, April 1992.

13. T. Moro et al., "Effects of Eight Weeks of Time-Restricted Feeding (16/8) on Basal Metabolism, Maximal Strength, Body Composition, Inflammation, and Cardiovascular Risk Factors in Resistance-Trained Males," *J Translational Med*, October 2016.

14. G. A. Thomas et al., "Immunoreactive and Bioactive Growth Hormone Responses to Resistance Exercise in Men Who Are Lean or Obese," *J Appl Physiology*, August 2011.

15. M. Khazaei et al., "New Findings on Biological Actions and Clinical Applications of Royal Jelly: A Review," *J Diet Suppl*, September 2018.

16. Y. Narita et al., "Effects of Long-Term Administration of Royal Jelly on Pituitary Weight and Gene Expression in Middle-Aged Female Rats," *Biosci Biotechnol Biochem*, February 2009.

17. I. Banerjee et al., "Growth Hormone Treatment and Cancer Risk," *Endocrinol Metab Clin North Am*, 2007.

18. R. Giordano et al., "Growth Hormone Treatment in Human Ageing: Benefits and Risks," *Hormones*, 2008.

19. T. L. Stanley and S. K. Grinspoon, "Effects of Growth Hormone-Releasing Hormone on Visceral Fat, Metabolic, and Cardiovascular Indices in Human Studies," *Growth Hormones IGF Res*, April 2015.

20. James Forsythe, *Anti-Aging Cures: Life Changing Secrets to Reverse the Effects of Aging* (New York: Vanguard Press, 2011), 31.

21. Forsythe, *Anti-Aging Cures*.

Chapter Eighteen: Andropause + Menopause = Couplepause

1. Jed Diamond, *The Irritable Male Syndrome: Managing the 4 Key Causes of Depression and Aggression* (Emmaus, PA: Rodale, 2004).

2. Tim Lott, "Yes, the Male Menopause DOES Exist—and It's Time Women Took It Seriously," *Daily Mail*, July 7, 2010, https://www.dailymail .co.uk/femail/article-1292604/Yes-male-menopause-DOES-exist--time -women-took-seriously.html (accessed 2/4/19).

3. E. A. Jannini and R. E. Nappi, "Couplepause: A New Paradigm in Treating Sexual Dysfunction during Menopause and Andropause," *Sexual Medicine Review*, January 2018.

4. Jannini and Nappi, "Couplepause."

5. H. W. Conaglen et al., "An Investigation of Sexual Dysfunction in Female Partners of Men with Erectile Dysfunction: How Interviews Expand on Questionnaire Responses," *Sex Relation Ther*, 2010.

6. J. Stephenson et al., "Before the Beginning: Nutrition and Lifestyle in the Preconception Period and Its Importance for Future Health," *Lancet*, May 2018.

7. T. P. Fleming et al., "Origins of Lifetime Health around the Time of Conception: Causes and Consequences," *Lancet*, May 2018.

8. M. Baker et al., "Intervention Strategies to Improve Nutrition and Health Behaviours before Conception," *Lancet*, May 2018.

9. M. A. Velazquez, T. Fleming, and A. J. Watkins, "Periconceptual Environment and the Developmental Origins of Disease," *Journal Endocrinology*, February 2019.

Bibliography

Achilli, C., et al. "Efficacy and Safety of Transdermal Testosterone in Post-menopausal Women with Hypoactive Sexual Desire Disorder: A Systematic Review and Meta-Analysis." *Fertility and Sterility*, February 2017.

Adler, R. A. "Management of Osteoporosis Inmen on Androgen Deprivation Therapy." *Maturitas*, February 2011.

Ajdzanovic, V. Z., et al. "Somatopause, Weaknesses of the Therapeutic Approaches and the Cautious Optimism Based on Experimental Ageing Studies with Soy Isoflavones." *EXCLI Journal*, March 2018.

Alibhai, S. M., et al. "Changes in Bone Mineral Density in Men Starting Androgen Deprivation Therapy and the Protective Role of Vitamin D." *Osteoporos International*, October 2013.

Andersen, M. L., et al. "The Association of Testosterone, Sleep, and Sexual Function in Men and Women." *Brain Research*, October 2011.

Anderson, C., and J. A. Horne. "A High Sugar Content, Low Caffeine Drink Does Not Alleviate Sleepiness but May Worsen It." *Human Psychopharmacology*, July 2006.

Antonio, L., et al. "Associations between Sex Steroids and the Development of Metabolic Syndrome: A Longitudinal Study in European Men." *Journal of Clinical Endocrinology and Metabolism*, April 2015.

Armanini, D., et al. "Licorice Consumption and Serum Testosterone in Healthy Man." *Experimental and Clinical Endocrinology and Diabetes*, September 2003.

Baas, W., and T. S. Kohler. "Testosterone Replacement Therapy and BPH/LUTS: What Is the Evidence?" *Current Urology Reports*, June 2016.

Bae, W. J., et al. "Antioxidant and Antifibrotic Effect of a Herbal Formulation in Vitro and in the Experimental Andropause Via Nrf2/HO-1 Signaling Pathway." *Oxidative Medicine and Cell Longevity*, 2017.

Bagley, Derek. "Growing Concerns: A Look at Growth Hormone Research." *Endocrine News*, July 2016.

Baker, L. D., et al. "Effects of Growth Hormone-Releasing Hormone on Cognitive Function in Adults with Mild Cognitive Impairment and Healthy Older Adults: Results of a Controlled Trial." *Archives of Neurology*, November 2012.

Baker, M., et al. "Intervention Strategies to Improve Nutrition and Health Behaviours before Conception." *Lancet*, May 2018.

Balliett, M., and J. R. Burke. "Changes in Anthropometric Measurements, Body Composition, Blood Pressure, Lipid Profile, and Testosterone in Patients Participating in a Low-Energy Dietary Intervention." *Journal of Chiropractic Medicine*, March 2013.

Banerjee, I., et al. "Growth Hormone Treatment and Cancer Risk." *Endocrinology and Metabolism Clinics of North America*, 2007.

Barake, M., et al. "Effects of Recombinant Human Growth Hormone Therapy on Bone Mineral Density in Adults with Growth Hormone Deficiency: A Meta-Analysis." *Journal of Clinical Endocrinology and Metabolism*, March 2014.

Basu, J., and S. Sharma. "Erectile Dysfunction Heralds Onset of Cardiovascular Disease." *Practitioner*, June 2016.

Baumann, G. P. "Growth Hormone Doping in Sports: A Critical Review of Use and Detection Strategies." *Endocrinology Review*, April 2012.

Beharry, S., and M. J. Heinrich. "Is the Hype around the Reproductive Health Claims of Maca (*Lepidium Meyenil Walp.*) Justified?" *Ethnopharmacology*, January 2018.

Belkoff, L., et al. "Efficacy and Safety of Testosterone Replacement Gel for Treating Hypogonadism in Men: Phase III Open-Label Studies." *Andrologia*, February 2018.

Bercea, R. M., et al. "Fatigue and Serum Testosterone in Obstructive Sleep Apnea Patients." *Clinical Respiratory Journal*, July 2015.

Bhasin, S., et al. "Effect of Testosterone Replacement on Measures of Mobility in Older Men with Mobility Limitation and Low Testosterone Concentrations: Secondary Analyses of the Testosterone Trials." *Lancet Diabetes Endrocinology*, November 2018.

Black, D. S., et al. "Mindfulness Meditation and Improvement in Sleep Quality and Daytime Impairment among Older Adults with Sleep Disturbances: A Randomized Clinical Trial." *Journal of the American Medical Association Internal Medicine*, 2015.

Blumenthal, J. A., et al. "Lifestyle and Neurocognition in Older Adults with Cognitive Impairments: A Randomized Trial." *Neurology*, December 2018.

Bluthgen, N. "Effects of the UV Filter Benzophenone-3 (Oxybenzone) at Low Concentrations in Zebrafish." *Toxicology and Applied Pharmacology*, September 2012.

Borst, S. E., et al. "Musculoskeletal and Prostate Effects of Combined Testosterone and Finasteride Administration in Older Hypogonadal Men: A Randomized Controlled Trial." *American Journal of Physiology, Endocrinology and Metabolism*, February 2014.

Bowden, A., et al. "Autogenic Training as a Behavioural Approach to Insomnia: A Prospective Study." *Primary Health Care Research & Development*, April 2012.

Brilla, L. R., et al. "Effects of a Novel Zinc-Magnesium Formulation on Hormones and Strength." *Journal of Exercise Physiology*, October 2000.

Brody, S. A., and D. L. Loriaux. "Epidemic of Gynecomastia among Haitian Refugees: Exposure to an Environmental Antiandrogen." *Endocrine Practice*, September 2003.

Brotzu, G., et al. "A Liposome-Based Formulation Containing Equol, Dihomo-Y-Linolenic Acid (DGLA), and Propionyl-L-Carnitine to Prevent and Treat Hair Loss: A Prospective Investigation." *Dermatologic Therapy*, October 2018.

Bursack, Carol Bradley. "Andropause: A Taboo Topic for Many Men." AgingCare.com. https://www.agingcare.com/articles/andropause-a-taboo -topic-for-many-men-197063.htm (accessed 2/4/19).

Burschtin, O., and J. Wang. "Testosterone Deficiency and Sleep Apnea." *Sleep Medicine Clinics*, December 2016.

Canguven, O., et al. "Vitamin D Treatment Improves Levels of Sexual Hormones, Metabolic Parameters and Erectile Function in Middle-Aged Vitamin D Deficient Men." *Aging Male*, March 2017.

Cao, H., et al. "Acupuncture for Treatment of Insomnia: A Systematic Review of Randomized Controlled Trials." *Journal of Alternative and Complementary Medicine*, 2009.

Carek, P. J., et al. "Exercise for the Treatment of Depression and Anxiety." *International Journal of Psychiatry Medicine*, 2011.

Carmacho, E. M. "Age-Associated Changes in Hypothalamic-Pituitary-Testicular Function in Middle-Aged and Older Men Are Modified by Weight Change and Lifestyle Factors: Longitudinal Results from the European Male Ageing Study." *European Journal of Endocrinology*, February 2013.

Caronia, L. M., et al. "Abrupt Decrease in Serum Testosterone Levels after an Oral Glucose Load in Men: Implications for Screening for Hypogonadism." *Clinical Endocrinology*, February 2013.

Carruthers, M., et al. "Evolution of Testosterone Treatment over 25 Years: Symptom Responses, Endocrine Profiles and Cardiovascular Changes." *Aging Male*, 2015.

Cheetham, T. C., et al. "Association of Testosterone Replacement with Cardiovascular Outcomes among Men with Androgen Deficiency." *Journal of the American Medical Association Internal Medicine*, April 2017.

Chen, C. Y., et al. "The Correlation between Emotional Distress and Aging Males' Symptoms at a Psychiatric Outpatient Clinic: Sexual Dysfunction as a Distinguishing Characteristic between Andropause and Anxiety/Depression in Aging Men." *Clinical Interventions in Aging*, 2013.

Chen, J., et al. "Antiandrogenic Properties of Parabens and Other Phenolic Containing Small Molecules in Personal Care Products." *Toxicology & Applied Pharmacology*, June 2017.

Chen, L., et al. "Sugar-Sweetened Beverage Intake and Serum Testosterone Levels in Adult Males 20–39 Years Old in the United States." *Reproductive Biology and Endocrinology*, June 2018.

Chen, M. L., et al. "The Effectiveness of Acupressure in Improving the Quality of Sleep of Institutionalized Residents." *Journal of Gerontology and Biological Science*, 1999.

Cherrier, M. M., et al. "Testosterone Supplementation Improves Spatial and Verbal Memory in Healthy Older Men." *Neurology*, July 2001.

Choi, K. T. "Botanical Characteristics, Pharmacological Effects and Medicinal Components of Korean Panax Ginseng CA Meyer." *Acta Parmacologica Sinica*, September 2008.

Choi, S. W., et al. "Effect of Korean Herbal Formula (Modified Ojayeon-jonghwan) on Androgen Receptor Expression in an Aging Rat Model of Late Onset Hypogonadism." *World Journal of Men's Health*, January 2019.

Choi, Y. D., et al. "Effects of Korean Ginseng Berry Extract on Sexual Function in Men with Erectile Dysfunction: A Multicenter, Placebo-Controlled, Double-Blind Clinical Study." *International Journal of Impotence Research*, March–April 2013.

Christudoss, P., et al. "Zinc Status of Patients with Benign Prostatic Hyperplasia and Prostate Carcinoma." *Indian Journal of Urology*, January–March 2011.

Clark, A. J., et al. "Onset of Impaired Sleep as a Predictor of Change in Health-Related Behaviours: Analyzing Observational Data as a Series of Non-Randomized Pseudo-Trials." *International Journal of Epidemiology*, June 2015.

Cleveland Clinic. "Bioidentical Hormones." www.clevelandclinic.org/health/articles/15660-bioidentical-hormones (accessed 1/22/19).

Conaglen, H. W., et al. "An Investigation of Sexual Dysfunction in Female Partners of Men with Erectile Dysfunction: How Interviews Expand on Questionnaire Responses." *Sexual Relations Therapy*, 2010.

Contreras, H. R., et al. "Testosterone Production and Spermatogenic Damage Induced by Organophosphorate Pesticides." *Biocell*, December 30, 2006.

Corona, G., et al. "Body Weight Loss Reverts Obesity-Associated Hypogonadotropic Hypogonadism: A Systematic Review and Meta-Analysis." *European Journal of Endocrinology*, May 2013.

———."Meta-Analysis of Results of Testosterone Therapy on Sexual Function Based on International Index of Erectile Function Scores." *European Urolology*, December 2017.

———. "Testosterone Supplementation and Body Composition: Results from a Meta-Analysis Study." *European Society of Endocrinology*, November 2015.

Courcoulas, A. P., et al. "Weight Change and Health Outcomes at 3 Years after Bariatric Surgery among Individuals with Severe Obesity." *Journal of the American Medical Association*, 2013.

Courtiss, E. H. "Gynecomastia: Analysis of 159 Patients and Current Recommendations for Treatment." *Plastic Reconstructive Surgery*, May 1987.

Crinnion, W. "Components of Practical Clinical Detox Programs—Sauna as a Therapeutic Tool." *Alternative Therapies in Health and Medicine*, March–April 2007.

Crinnion, W. J. "Sauna as a Valuable Clinical Tool for Cardiovascular, Autoimmune, Toxicant-Induced and Other Chronic Health Problems." *Alternative Medicine Review*, September 2011.

Cui, D., et al. "The Effect of Chronic Prostatitis on Zinc Concentration of Prostatic Fluid and Seminal Plasma: A Systematic Review and Meta-Analysis." *Current Medical Research and Opinion*, 2015.

Cui, Y., and Y. Zhang. "The Effect of Androgen-Replacement Therapy on Prostate Growth: A Systematic Review and Meta-Analysis." *European Urology*, November 2013.

Cunningham, G. R., et al. "Association of Sex Hormones with Sexual Function, Vitality, and Physical Function of Symptomatic Older Men with Low Testosterone Levels at Baseline in the Testosterone Trials." *Journal of Clinical Endocrinology Metabolism*, March 2015.

———. "Testosterone Treatment and Sexual Function in Older Men with Low Testosterone Levels." *Journal of Clinical Endocrinology Metabolism*, August 2016.

Cutler, Winifred. *Love Cycles: The Science of Intimacy*. New York: Random House, 1995.

Damiano, R., et al. "The Role of Cucurbita Pepo in the Management of Patients Affected by Lower Urinary Tract Symptoms Due to Benign Prostatic Hyperplasia: A Narrative Review." *Archivio Italiano Urologia Andrologia*, July 2016.

Daniel, J. M., et al. "The Critical Period Hypothesis of Estrogen Effect on Cognition: Insights From Basic Research." *Biochimica et Biphysica Acta*, 2010.

Datta, K., et al. "Eclipa Alba Extract with Potential for Hair Growth Promoting Activity." *Journal of Ethnopharmacology*, July 2009.

De Andrade, E., et al. "Study of the Efficacy of Korean Red Ginseng in the Treatment of Erectile Dysfunction." *Asian Journal of Andrology*, March 2007.

De La Iglesia, R., et al. "Dietary Strategies Implicated in the Prevention and Treatment of Metabolic Syndrome." *International Journal of Molecular Science*, November 2016.

Debruyne, F. M., et al. "Testosterone Treatment Is Not Associated with Increased Risk of Prostate Cancer or Worsening of Lower Urinary Tract Symptoms: Prostate Health Outcomes in the Registry of Hypogonadism in Men." *BJU Int*, February 2017.

Del Fabbro, E., et al. "Testosterone Replacement for Fatigue in Hypgonadal Ambulatory Males with Advanced Cancer: A Preliminary Double-Blind Placebo-Controlled Trial." *Support Care Cancer*, September 2013.

Delay, K. J., and T. S. Kohler. "Testosterone and the Prostate: Artifacts and Truths." *Urological Clinics of North America*, August 2016.

Della Camera, P. A., et al. "Sexual Health, Adherence to Mediterranean Diet, Body Weight, Physical Activity and Mental State: Factors Correlated to Each Other." *Urologia*, October 2017.

Di Luigi, L., et al. "Prevalence of Undiagnosed Testosterone Deficiency in Aging Athletes: Does Exercise Training Influence the Symptoms of Male Hypogonadism?" *Journal of Sexual Medicine*, July 2010.

Diamond, Jed. "What Your Doctor Won't Tell You about Male Hormonal Cycles." Goodtherapy.org, October 9, 2012. https://www.goodtherapy .org/blog/male-hormonal-cycles-andropause-1009127 (accessed 2/16/19).

Diamond, Jed. *The Irritable Male Syndrome: Managing the 4 Key Causes of Depression and Aggression.* Emmaus, PA: Rodale, 2004.

Dibaba, D. T., et al. "Dietary Magnesium Intake and Risk of Metabolic Syndrome: A Meta-Analysis." *Diabetes Medicine*, November 2014.

Ding, E. L., et al. "Sex Differences of Endogenous Ex Hormones and Risk of Type 2 Diabetes: A Systematic Review and Meta-Analysis." *Journal of the American Medical Association*, March 2006.

Dobs, A., and M. J. Darkes. "Incidence and Management of Gynecomastia in Men Treated for Prostate Cancer." *Journal of Urology*, November 2005.

Ebert, S. M., et al. "Identification and Small Molecule Inhibition of an Activating Transcription Factor 4 (ATF4)-Dependent Pathway to Age-Related Skeletal Muscle Weakness and Atrophy." *Journal of Biological Chemistry*, October 2015.

Eichholzer, M., et al. "Serum Sex Steroids Hormones and Frailty in Older American Men of the Third National Health and Nutrition Examination Survey." *Aging Male*, December 2012.

Eisenberg, M. L. "Testosterone Replacement Therapy and Prostate Cancer Incidence." *World Journal of Men's Health*, December 2015.

Epstein, Samuel, and Randall Fitzgerald. *Toxic Beauty: How Cosmetics and Personal-Care Products Endanger Your Health*. Dallas, TX: Benbella, 2009.

Esposito, K., et al. "Dietary Factors, Mediterranean Diet and Erectile Dysfunction." *Journal of Sex Medicine*, July 2010.

Eziefula, C. U., et al. "You Know I've Joined Your Club . . . I'm in the Hot Flush Boy: A Qualitative Exploration of Hot Flashes and Night Sweats in Men Undergoing Androgen Deprivation Therapy for Prostate Cancer." *Psycho-oncology*, December 2013.

Ezzati, M., et al. "Trends in Adult Body-Mass Index in 200 Countries from 1975 to 2014: A Pooled Analysis of 1,698 Population-Based Measurement Studies with 19.2 Million Participants." *Lancet*, April 2016.

Fallah, A., et al. "Zinc Is an Essential Element for Male Fertility: A Review of Zn Roles in Men's Health, Germination, Sperm Quality, and Fertilization." *Journal of Reproduction and Infertility*, April–June 2018.

Finkelstein, J. S., et al. "Gonadal Steroids and Body Composition, Strength, and Sexual Function in Men." *New England Journal of Medicine*, September 2013.

Fleming, T. P., et al. "Origins of Lifetime Health around the Time of Conception: Causes and Consequences." *Lancet*, May 2018.

Ford, A. H., et al. "Sex Hormones and Incident Dementia in Older Men: The Health in Men Study." *Psychoneuroendocrinology*, September 2018.

Forsythe, James. *Anti-Aging Cures: Life Changing Secrets to Reverse the Effects of Aging*. New York: Vanguard Press, 2011.

Frederick, D. W., et al. "Loss of NAD Homeostasis Leads to Progressive and Reversible Degeneration of Skeletal Muscle." *Cell Metabolism*, August 2016.

Frederiksen, L., et al. "Testosterone Therapy Increased Muscle Mass and Lipid Oxidation in Aging Men." *Age*, February 2012.

Fryar, C. D., et al. "Fast Food Consumption among Adults in the United States, 2013–2016." *NCHS Data Brief*, no. 322, October 2018.

Fujiwara, Y., et al. "Hearing Laughter Improves the Recovery Process of the Autonomic Nervous System after a Stress-Loading Task: A Randomized Controlled Trial." *Biopsychosocial Medicine*, December 2018.

Fuller, S. J., et al. "Androgens in the Etiology of Alzheimer's Disease in Aging Men and Possible Therapeutic Interventions." *Journal of Alzheimer's Disease*, September 2007.

Gardener, S. L., and S. R. Rainey-Smith. "The Role of Nutrition in Cognitive Function and Brain Ageing in the Elderly." *Current Nutrition Reports*, September 2018.

Gaudriault, P., et al. "Endocrine Disruption in Human Fetal Testis Explants by Individual and Combined Exposures to Selected Pharmaceuticals, Pesticides, and Environmental Pollutants." *Environtal Health Perspectives*, August 2017.

Genuis, S. J., et al. "Human Excretion of Bisphenol A: Blood, Urine, Sweat Study." *Journal of Environmental Public Health*, 2012.

George, A., and R. Henkel. "Phytoandrogenic Properties of Eurycoma Longifolia as Natural Alternative to Testosterone Replacement Therapy." *Andrologia*, September 2014.

Giordano, R., et al. "Growth Hormone Treatment in Human Ageing: Benefits and Risks." *Hormones*, 2008.

Giugliano, F., et al. "Adherence to Mediterranean Diet and Erectile Dysfunction in Men with Type 2 Diabetes." *Journal of Sexual Medicine*, May 2010.

Glaser, R., and C. Dimitrakakis. "Testosterone Therapy in Women: Myths and Misconceptions." *Maturitas*, 2013.

Golds, G., et al. "Male Hypogonadism and Osteoporosis: The Effects, Clinical Consequences, and Treatment of Testosterone Deficiency in Bone Health." *International Journal of Endocrinology*, 2017.

Golla, V., and A. L. Kaplan. "Testosterone Therapy on Active Surveillance and Following Definitive Treatment for Prostate Cancer." *Current Urology Reports*, July 2017.

Gonzales, G. F., et al. "Effect of *Lepidium meyenii* (Maca), a Root with Aphrodisiac and Fertility-Enhancing Properties, on Serum Reproductive Hormone Levels in Adult Healthy Men." *Journal of Endocrinology*, January 2003.

Gonzalez, A., et al. "Zinc Intake from Supplements and Diet and Prostate Cancer." *Nutrition and Cancer*, 2009.

Gouveia, M., et al. "The Role of Testosterone in the Improvement of Sexual Desire in Postmenopausal Women: An Evidence-Based Clinical Review." *Acta Medica Portuguesa*, November 2018.

Grindler, N. M., et al. "Persistent Organic Pollutants and Early Menopause in U. S. Women." *PLOS One,* January 2015.

Gruenwald, I., et al. "Shockwave Treatment of Erectile Dysfunction." *Therapeutic Advances in Urology*, April 2013.

Gu, Y., et al. "Mediterranean Diet and Brain Structure in a Multiethnic Elderly Cohort." *Neurology*, October 2015.

Gudelin, H. W., et al. "A Randomized, Active- and Placebo-Controlled Study of the Efficacy and Safety of Different Doses of Dutasteride versus Placebo and Finasteride in the Treatment of Male Subjects with Androgenetic Alopecia." *Journal of the American Academy of Dermatology*, March 2014.

Hackney, A. C. "Effects of Endurance Exercise on the Reproductive System of Men: The 'Exercise-Hypogonadal Male Condition.'" *Journal of Endocrinological Investigation*, October 2008.

Haider, A., et al. "Hypogonadal Obese Men with and without Diabetes Mellitus Type 2 Lose Weight and Show Improvement in Cardiovascular Risk Factors When Treated with Testosterone: An Observational Study." *Obesity Research and Clinical Practice*, July–August 2014.

Hannuksela, M. L., et al. "Benefits and Risks of Sauna Bathing." *American Journal of Medicine*, February 2001.

Hardman, R. J., et al. "Adherence to a Mediterranean-Style Diet and Effects on Cognition in Adults: A Qualitative Evaluation and Systematic Review of Longitudinal and Prospective Trials." *Frontiers in Nutrition*, July 2016.

Hartman, M. L., et al. "Augmented Growth Hormone (GH) Secretory Burst Frequency and Amplitude Mediate Enhanced GH Secretion during a Two-Day Fast in Normal Men." *Journal of Clinical Endocrinology and Metabolism*, April 1992.

Harvard Health Publishing. "Testosterone, Prostate Cancer, and Balding: Is There a Link?" January 23, 2017. https://www.health.harvard.edu/mens-health/testosterone-prostate-cancer-and-balding-is-there-a-link-thefamilyhealth-guide (accessed 11/11/18).

Harvey, A. G., and S. Payne. "The Management of Unwanted Pre-Sleep Thoughts in Insomnia: Distraction with Imagery versus General Distraction." *Behaviour Research and Therapy*, March 2002.

Hauser, R., et al. "Male Reproductive Disorders, Diseases, and Costs of Exposure to Endocrine-Disrupting Chemicals in the European Union." *Journal of Clinical Endocrinology and Metabolism*, April 2015.

Heidari, R., et al. "Can Testosterone Level Be a Good Predictor of Late-Onset Hypogonadism?" *Andrologia*, May 2015.

Heindel, J. J., et al. "Endocrine Disruptors and Obesity." *National Review of Endocrinology*, November 2015.

Herbst, K. L., et al. "Testosterone Action on Skeletal Muscle." *Current Opinion in Clinical Nutrition and Metabolic Care*, May 2004.

Hines, S. L., et al. "The Role of Mammography in Male Patients with Breast Symptoms." *Mayo Clinic Proceedings*, 2007.

Hirokawa, K., et al. "Job Demands as a Potential Modifier of the Association between Testosterone Deficiency and Andropause Symptoms in Japanese Middle-Aged Workers: A Cross-Sectional Study." *Maturitas*, November 2012.

———. "Modification Effects of Changes in Job Demands on Associations between Changes in Testosterone Levels and Andropause Symptoms: 2-Year Follow-Up Study in Male Middle-Aged Japanese Workers." *International Journal of Behavior Medicine*, August 2016.

Hirsh, S., et al. "An Open Label Study to Evaluate the Effect of *Kaempferia parviflora* in Support of Erectile Function and Male Sexual Health among Overall Healthy Males 50–70." *FASEB Journal*, April 2017.

Holtorf, K. "The Bioidentical Hormone Debate: Are Bioidentical Hormones (Estradiol, Estriol, and Progesterone) Safer or More Efficacious Than Commonly Used Synthetic Versions in Hormone Replacement Therapy?" *Postgraduate Medical Journal*, January 2009.

Hong, B., et al. "A Double-Blind Crossover Study Evaluating the Efficacy of Korean Red Ginseng in Patients with Erectile Dysfunction: A Preliminary Report." *Journal of Urolology*, November 2002.

Howatson, G., et al. "Effect of Tart Cherry Juice (*Prunus cerasus*) on Melatonin Levels and Enhanced Sleep Quality." *European Journal of Nutrition*, December 2012.

Hu, H., et al. "Racial Differences in Age-Related Variations of Testosterone Levels among US Males: Potential Implications for Prostate Cancer and Personalized Medication." *Journal of Racial and Ethnic Health Disparities*, March 2015.

Hua, J. T., et al. "Effects of Testosterone Therapy on Cognitive Function in Aging: A Systematic Review." *Cognitive and Behavioral Neurology*, September 2016.

Huhtaniemi, I. T. "Andropause—Lessons from the European Male Ageing Study." *Annals of Endocrinology*, May 2014.

Hung, S. K., et al. "The Effectiveness and Efficacy of *Rhodiola Rosea L*: A Systematic Review of Randomized Clinical Trials." *Phytomedicine*, February 2011.

Jackson, G., et al. "The Assessment of Vascular Risk in Men with Erectile Dysfunction: The Role of the Cardiologist and General Physician." *International Journal of Clinical Practice*, November 2013.

Jacobs, G. D. "Clinical Applications of the Relaxation Response and Mind-Body Interventions." *Journal of Alternative and Complementary Medicine*, 2001.

Jakiel, G., et al. "Andropause—State of the Art 2015 and Review of Selected Aspects." *Menopause Review*, March 2015.

Jang, D. J., et al. "Red Ginseng for Treating Erectile Dysfunction: A Systematic Review." *British Journal of Clinical Pharmacology*, October 2008.

Janiszewska, M., et al. "Men's Knowledge about Osteoporosis and Its Risk Factors." *Przeglad Menopauzalny*, November 2016.

Jannini, E. A., and R. E. Nappi. "Couplepause: A New Paradigm in Treating Sexual Dysfunction during Menopause and Andropause." *Sexual Medicine Review*, January 2018.

Janson, Kenneth. "Benefits of Hormone Replacement Therapy." *Previentmd*, 2016. www.myhealthengage.com (accessed 1/31/19).

———. "Decreasing the Risk of Cognitive Decline." *Previentmd*. http://myhealthengage.com/blogs/view/220/decreasing-the-risk-of-cognitive-decline (accessed 1/25/19).

Jaruvongvanich, V., et al. "Testosterone, Sex Hormone–Binding Globulin and Nonalcoholic Fatty Liver Disease: A Systematic Review and Meta-Analysis." *Annals of Hepatology*, May 2017.

Johnson, R. E., and H. Murad. "Gynecomastia: Pathophysiology, Evaluation, and Management." *Mayo Clinic Proceedings*, November 2009.

Jones, T. H., and D. M. Kelly. "Randomized Controlled Trials—Mechanistic Studies of Testosterone and the Cardiovascular System." *Asian Journal of Andrology*, March–April 2018.

Kalman, D. S., and S. J. Hewlings. "The Effects of Morus Alba and Acacia Catechu on Quality of Life and Overall Function in Adults with Osteoarthritis of the Knee." *Journal of Nutrition and Metabolism*, 2017.

Kang, J. L., et al. "Promotion Effect of Schisandra Nigra on the Growth of Hair." *European Journal of Dermatology*, March–April 2009.

Karemer, W. J., et al. "Hormonal Responses and Adaptations to Resistance Exercise and Training." *Sports Medcine*, 2005.

Kelishadi, R., et al. "Role of Environmental Chemicals in Obesity: A Systematic Review on the Current Evidence." *Journal of Environmental and Public Health*, 2013.

Khazaei, M., et al. "New Findings on Biological Actions and Clinical Applications of Royal Jelly: A Review." *Journal of Dietary Supplements*, September 2018.

Khera, M. "Testosterone Therapy for Female Sexual Dysfunction." *Sexual Medicine Review*, 2015.

Khera, M., et al. "Improved Sexual Function with Testosterone Replacement Therapy in Hypogonadal Men: Real-World Data from the Testim Registry in the United States." *Journal of Sexual Medicine*, November 2011.

Khoo, J., et al. "Comparing Effects of Low- and High-Volume Moderate-Intensity Exercise on Sexual Function and Testosterone in Obese Men." *Journal of Sexual Medicine*, July 2013.

Khosravi, S., et al. "Are Andropause Symptoms Related to Depression?" *Aging Clinical and Experimental Research*, December 2015.

Khusid, M. A., et al. "The Emerging Role of Mindfulness Meditation as Effective Self-Management Strategy, Part 1: Clinical Implications for Depression, Post-Traumatic Stress Disorder, and Anxiety." *Military Medicine*, September 2016.

Kim, S. C. "Promotion Effect of Norgalanthamine, a Component of Crinum Asiaticum, on Hair Growth." *European Journal of Dermatology*, January–February 2010.

Kim, S. D., and K. S. Cho. "Obstructive Sleep Apnea and Testosterone Deficiency." *World Journal of Men's Health*, January 2019.

Kim, S. H., et al. "Laughter and Stress Relief in Cancer Patients: A Pilot Study." *Evidence-Based Complementary and Alternative Medicine*, 2015.

Klap, J., et al. "The Relationship between Total Testosterone Levels and Prostate Cancer: A Review of the Continuing Controversy." *Journal of Urology*, February 2015.

Kocaadam, B., et al. "Curcumin, an Active Component of Turmeric (*Curcuma longa*), and Its Effects on Health." *Critical Review of Food Science and Nutrition*, 2017.

Koehler, K., et al. "Serum Testosterone and Urinary Excretion of Steroid Hormone Metabolites after Administration of a High Dose Zinc Supplement." *European Journal of Clinical Nutrition*, 2009.

Kohn, T. P., et al. "Effects of Testosterone Replacement Therapy on Lower Urinary Tract Symptoms: A Systematic Review and Meta-analysis." *European Urolology*, June 2016.

Komer, Lawrence D. "Andropause: Roy's Story." Komer Health Centre. http://komer-womens-health.com/male-menopause/ (accessed 2/16/19).

Kotirum, S., et al. "Efficacy of Tongkat Ali (*Eurycoma longifolia*) on Erectile Function Improvement: Systematic Review and Meta-analysis of Randomized Controlled Trials." *Complementary Therapies in Medicine*, October 2015.

Kovac, J. R., et al. "Dietary Adjuncts for Improving Testosterone Levels in Hypogonadal Males." *American Journal of Men's Health*, August 2015.

Kraemer, W. J., et al. "Effects of Heavy-Resistance Training on Hormonal Response Patterns in Younger vs. Older Men." *Journal of Applied Physiology*, September 1999.

Kvam, S., et al. "Exercise as a Treatment for Depression: A Meta-analysis." *Journal of Affective Disorders*, September 2016.

Lashkari, M., et al. "Association of Serum Testosterone and Dehydroepian-drosterone Sulfate with Rheumatoid Arthritis: A Case Control Study." *Electronic Physician*, March 2018.

Laughlin, G. A., et al. "Low Serum Testosterone and Mortality in Older Men." *Journal of Clinical Endocrinology and Metabolism*, January 2008.

Lee, C., et al. "The Prevalence and Correlates of the Positive Androgen Deficiency in the Aging Male (ADAM) Questionnaire among Psychiatric Outpatients: A Cross-Sectional Survey of 176 Men in a General Hospital in Taiwan." *Neuropsychiatric Disease Treatment*, January 2015.

Lee, K. W., et al. "A Randomized, Controlled Study of Treatment with Ojayeonjonghwan for Patients with Late Onset Hypogonadism." *Aging Male*, July 2018.

Lee, S. G., et al. "Panax Ginseng Leaf Extracts Exert Anti-obesity Effects in High-Fat-Diet-Induced Obese Rats." *Nutrients*, September 2017.

Lerchbaum, E., et al. "Effects of Vitamin D Supplementation on Androgens in Men with Low Testosterone Levels: A Randomized Controlled Trial." *European Journal of Nutrition*, November 2018.

Lin, L., et al. "The Effects of a Modified Mindfulness-Based Stress Reduction Program for Nurses: A Randomized Controlled Trial." *Workplace Health*, October 2018.

Lincoln, G. A. "The Irritable Male Syndrome." *Reproduction, Fertility and Development*, 2001.

Liu, G., et al. "Efficacy and Safety of MMFS-01, a Synapse Density Enhancer, for Treating Cognitive Impairment in Older Adults: A Randomized, Double-Blind, Placebo-Controlled Trial." *Journal of Alzheimer's Disease*, 2016.

Liu, T. C., et al. "Effect of Acute DHEA Administration on Free Testosterone in Middle-Aged and Young Men Following High-Intensity Interval Training." *European Journal of Applied Physiology*, July 2013.

Loeb, S., et al. "Testosterone Replacement Therapy and Risk of Favorable and Aggressive Prostate Cancer." *Journal of Clinical Oncology*, May 2017.

Lopez, D. S. "Racial/Ethnic Differences in Serum Sex Steroid Hormone Concentrations in US Adolescent Males." *Cancer Causes Control*, April 2013.

Lott, Tim. "Yes, the Male Menopause DOES Exist—and It's Time Women Took It Seriously." *Daily Mail*, July 7, 2010. https://www.dailymail.co.uk/femail/article-1292604/yes-male-menopause-does-exist--time-women-took-seriously.html (accessed 2/4/19).

Luboshitzky, R., et al. "Disruption of the Nocturnal Testosterone Rhythm by Sleep Fragmentation in Normal Men." *Journal of Clinical Endorcinology and Metabolism*, March 2001.

Lucas, M., et al. "Inflammatory Dietary Pattern and Risk of Depression among Women." *Brain, Behavior, and Immunity*, February 2014.

Luo, Y., et al "Sex Hormones Predict the Incidence of Erectile Dysfunction: From a Population-Based Prospective Cohort Study (FAMHES)." *Journal of Sexual Medicine*, May 2015.

Luthy, K. B., and C. Williams. "Comparison of Testosterone Replacement Therapy Medications for Treatment of Hypogonadism." *Journal of Nurse Practitioners*, 2017.

Madaeva, I. M., et al. "Obstructive Sleep Apnea Syndrome and Age-Related Hypogonadism." *Zhurnal Nevrologii i Psikhiatrii Imeni S S. Korsakova*, 2017.

Maggio, M., et al. "The Hormonal Pathway to Cognitive Impairment in Older Men." *Journal of Nutrition, Health and Aging*, 2012.

Maheshwari, A., et al. "Efficacy of Furosap, a Novel Trigonella Foenum-Graecum Seed Extract, in Enhancing Testosterone Level and Improving Sperm Profile in Male Volunteers." *International Journal of Medical Science*, January 2017.

Mahmoud, A. M., et al. "Zinc Intake and Risk of Prostate Cancer: Case-Control Study and Meta-analysis." *PLOS One*, November 2016.

Malinowski, P., et al. "Mindful Aging: The Effects of Regular Brief Mindfulness Practice on Electrophysiological Markers of Cognitive and Affective Processing in Older Adults." *Mindfulness*, December 2015.

Mannu, G. S., et al. "Role of Tamoxifen in Idiopathic Gynecomastia: A 10-Year Prospective Cohort Study." *Breast Journal*, November 2018.

Marks, L. S., et al. "Effects of a Saw Palmetto Herbal Blend in Men with Symptomatic Benign Prostatic Hyperplasia." *Journal of Urology*, May 2000.

Martina, V., et al. "Short-Term Dehydroepiandrosterone Treatment Increases Platelet cGMP Production in Elderly Male Subjects." *Clinical Endocrinology (Oxf)*, March 2006.

Martinez, J., and J. E. Lewi. "An Unusual Case of Gynecomastia Associated with Soy Product Consumption." *Endocrin Practice*, May–June 2008.

Masuda, A., et al. "The Effects of Repeated Thermal Therapy for Two Patients with Chronic Fatigue Syndrome." *Journal of Psychosomatic Research*, April 2005.

Matousek, R. H., and B. B. Sherwin. "Sex Steroid Hormones and Cognitive Functioning in Healthy, Older Men." *Hormones and Behavior*, March 2010.

Maughan, R. J. "Impact of Mild Dehydration on Wellness and on Exercise Performance." *European Journal of Clinical Nutrition*, December 2003.

Mayo Clinic. "Benign Prostatic Hyperplasia: Overview." https://www.mayo clinic.org/diseases-conditions/benign-prostatic-hyperplasia/symptoms -causes/syc-20370087 (accessed 1/18/19).

———."Bioidentical Hormones: Are They Safer?" https://www.mayo clinic.org/diseases-conditions/menopause/expert-answers/bioidentical -hormones/faq-20058460 (accessed 1/22/19).

———. "Enlarged Breasts in Men (Gynecomastia): Overview." https:// www.mayoclinic.org (accessed 1/12/19).

———. "Prostatitis: Overview." https://www.mayoclinic.org/diseases -conditions/prostatitis/symptoms-causes/syc-20355766 (accessed 1/19/19).

McHenry, J., et al. "Sex Differences in Anxiety and Depression: Role of Testosterone." *Frontiers in Neuroendocrinology*, January 2014.

McNicholas, T., and T. Ong. "Review of Testim Gel." *Expert Opinion on Pharmacotherapy*, March 2016.

Mediakovic, S., et al. "Effect of Nonpersistent Pesticides on Estrogen Receptor, Androgen Receptor, and Aryl Hydrocarbon Receptor." *Environmental Toxicology*, October 2014.

Meeker, J. D., et al. "House Dust Concentrations of Organophosphate Flame Retardants in Relation to Hormone Levels and Semen Quality Parameters." *Environmental Health Perspectives*, March 2010.

Mekala, K. C., and N. A. Tritos. "Effects of Recombinant Human Growth Hormone Therapy in Obesity in Adults: A Meta Analysis." *Journal of Clinical Endocrinology and Metabolism*, January 2009.

Miller, J. W., et al. "Vitamin D Status and Rates of Cognitive Decline in a Multiethnic Cohort of Older Adults." *Journal of the American Medical Association Neurology*, November 2015.

Milner, C. E., and K. Cote. "Benefits of Napping in Healthy Adults: Impact of Nap Length, Time of Day, Age, and Experience with Napping." *Journal of Sleep Research*, May 2009.

Min-Ji, B., et al. "Safety of Red Ginseng Oil for Single Oral Administration in Sprague-Dawley Rats." *Journal of Ginseng Research*, January 2014.

Moffat, S. D., et al. "Longitudinal Assessment of Serum Free Testosterone Concentration Predicts Memory Performance and Cognitive Status in Elderly Men." *Journal of Clinical Endcrinology and Metabolism*, November 2002.

Mohammed, O., et al. "The Quantitative ADAM Questionnaire: A New Tool in Quantifying the Severity of Hypogonadism." *International Journal of Impotence Research*, January 2010.

Molendijk, M., et al. "Diet Quality and Depression Risk: A Systematic Review and Dose-Response Meta-Analysis of Prospective Studies." *Journal of Affective Disorders*, January 2018.

Morales, A., et al. "Androgens and Sexual Function: A Placebo-Controlled, Randomized, Double-Blind Study of Testosterone vs. Dehydroepiandrosterone in Men with Sexual Dysfunction and Androgen Deficiency." *Aging Male*, December 2009.

Moran, L. J., et al. "Long-Term Effects of a Randomised Controlled Trial Comparing High Protein or High Carbohydrate Weight Loss Diets on Testosterone, SHBG, Erectile and Urinary Function in Overweight and Obese Men." *PLOS One*, September 2016.

Morgentaler, A. "Testosterone, Cardiovascular Risk, and Hormonophobia." *Journal of Sexual Medicine*, 2014.

Morley, J. E., et al. "Validation of a Screening Questionnaire for Androgen Deficiency in Aging Males." *Metabolism*, 2000.

Moro, T., et al. "Effects of Eight Weeks of Time-Restricted Feeding (16/8) on Basal Metabolism, Maximal Strength, Body Composition, Inflammation, and Cardiovascular Risk Factors in Resistance-Trained Males." *Journal of Translational Medicine*, October 2016.

Morris, M. C., et al. "MIND Diet Slows Cognitive Decline with Aging." *Alzheimer's and Dementia*, September 2015.

Mulligan, I., et al. "Growth Hormone Doping: A Review." *Open Access Journal of Sports Medicine*, July 2011.

Myhill, S., et al. "Targeting Mitochrondrial Dysfunction in the Treatment of Myalgic Encephalomyelitis/Chronic Fatigue Syndrome: A Clinical Audit." *International Journal of Clinical and Experimental Medicine*, 2013.

Nahata, A., et al. "Ameliorative Effects of Stinging Nettled (*Urtica dioica*) on Testosterone-Induced Prostatic Hyperplasia in Rats." *Andrologia*, May 2012.

Narita, Y., et al. "Effects of Long-Term Administration of Royal Jelly on Pituitary Weight and Gene Expression in Middle-Aged Female Rats." *Bioscience Biotechnology and Biochemistry*, February 2009.

National Center for Complementary and Integrative Health. "What the Science Says about the Effectiveness of St. John's Wort for Depression." https://nccih.nih.gov/health/stjohnswort/sjw-and-depression.htm.

National Institute of Diabetes and Digestive and Kidney Diseases. "Types of Bariatric Surgery." https://www.niddk.nih.gov/health-information/weight-management/bariatric-surgery/types (accessed 1/14/19).

National Sleep Foundation. "Cognitive Behavioral Therapy for Insomnia." https://www.sleepfoundation.org/sleep-news/cognitive-behavioral-therapy-insomnia (accessed 1/4/19).

Nave, G., et al. "Single Dose Testosterone Administration Impairs Cognitive Reflection in Men." *Psychological Science*, October 2017.

———. "Single-Dose Testosterone Administration Increases Men's Preference for Status Goods." *Nature Communications*, 2018.

Nery, S. F., et al. "Mindfulness-Based Program for Stress Reduction in Infertile Women: Randomized Controlled Trial." *Stress Health*, October 2018.

Neychev, V., and V. Mitev. "Pro-Sexual and Androgen Enhancing Effects of *Tribulus terrestris L.*: Fact or Fiction." *Journal of Ethnopharmacology*, February 2016.

Nikkola, Tom. "Irritable Male Syndrome, Andropause, and Reclaiming Your Manhood." *Tomnikkola Newsletter*. https://tomnikkola.com/irritable -male-syndrome-andropause-manhood/ (accessed 2/16/19).

Oi, Y., et al. "Garlic Supplementation Increases Testicular Testosterone and Decreases Plasma Corticosterone in Rats Fed a High Protein Diet." *Journal of Nutrition*, August 2001.

Okada, K., et al. "Improved Lower Urinary Tract Symptoms Associated with Testosterone Replacement Therapy in Japanese Men with Late-Onset Hypogonadism." *American Journal of Men's Health*, June 2016.

Olsen, E. A., et al. "The Importance of Dual 5x-Reductase Inhibition in the Treatment of Male Pattern Hair Loss: Results of a Randomized Placebo-Controlled Study of Dutasteride versus Finasteride." *Journal of the American Academy of Dermatology*, December 2006.

Ooi, S. L., and S. C. Pak. "Serenoa Repens for Lower Urinary Tract Symptoms/Benign Prostatic Hyperplasia: Current Evidence and Its Clinical Implications in Naturopathic Medicine." *Journal of Alternative and Complementary Medicine*, August 2017.

Orton, F., et al. "Widely Used Pesticides with Previously Unknown Endocrine Activity Revealed as in Vitro Antiandrogens." *Environmental Health Perspectives*, June 2011.

Palisin, T. E., and J. J. Stacy. "Ginseng: Is It in the Root?" *Current Sports Medicine Reports*, June 2006.

Paller, C. J., et al. "Relationship of Sex Steroid Hormones with Bone Mineral Density (BMD) in a Nationally Representative Sample of Men." *Clinical Endocrinology*, January 2009.

Pandit, S., et al. "Clinical Evaluation of Purified Shilajit on Testosterone Levels in Healthy Volunteers." *Andrologia*, January 2016.

Pascoe, M. C., et al. "Yoga, Mindfulness-Based Stress Reduction and Stress-Related Physiological Measures: A Meta-analysis." *Psychoneuroendocrinology*, December 2017.

Pearl, J. A., et al. "Testosterone Supplementation Does Not Worsen Urinary Tract Symptoms." *Journal of Urolology*, November 2013.

Pelling, Rowan. "Watching the Male Menopause in Action Isn't Pretty." *Telegraph-UK*, July 30, 2015. https://www.telegraph.co.uk/men/active/mens-health/11774259/watching-the-male-menopause-in-action-isnt-pretty.html (accessed 2/16/19).

Pikwer, M., et al. "Association between Testosterone Levels and Risk of Future Rheumatoid Arthritis in Men: A Population-Based Case-Control Study." *Annals of the Rheumatoid Disease*, March 2014.

Prado, A. C., and P. F. Castillo. "Minimal Surgical Access to Treat Gynecomastia with the Use of a Power-Assisted Arthroscopic-Endoscopic Cartilage Shaver." *Plastic Reconstrive Surgery*, March 2005.

Pratte, M. A., et al. "An Alternative Treatment for Anxiety: A Systematic Review of Human Trial Results Reported for the Ayurvedic Herb Ashwagandha (*Withania somnifera*)." *Journal of Alternative and Complementary Medicine*, December 2014.

Preuss, H. G., et al. "Randomized Trial of a Combination of Natural Products (Cernitin, Saw Palmetto, B-Sitosterol, Vitamin E) on Symptoms of Benign Prostatic Hyperplasia (BPH)." *International Urology and Nephrology*, 2001.

Purohit, V. "Can Alcohol Promote Aromatization of Androgens to Estrogens? A Review." *Alcohol*, November 2000.

Pye, S. R., et al. "Late-Onset Hypogonadism and Mortality in Aging Men." *Journal of Clinical Endocrinology and Metabolism*, April 2014.

Rabijewski, M., et al. "Hormonal Determinants of the Severity of Andropausal and Depressive Symptoms in Middle-Aged and Elderly Men with Prediabetes." *Clinical Interventions in Aging*, August 2015.

Rafiq, R., et al. "Associations of Different Body Fat Deposits with Serum 25-Hydroxyvitamin D Concentrations." *European Society of Endocrinology*, 2018.

Rao, A., et al. "Testofen, a Specialized Trigonella Foenum-Graecum Seed Extract Reduces Age-Related Symptoms of Androgen Decrease, Increases Testosterone Levels and Improves Sexual Function in Healthy Aging Males in a Double-Blind Randomized Clinical Study." *Aging Male*, June 2016.

Reiter, K. "Improved Cardiorespiratory Fitness Is Associated with Increased Cortical Thickness in Mild Cognitive Impairment." *Journal of the International Neuropsychological Society*, 2015.

Reviews.com. "The Best Testosterone Booster." www.reviews.com/testosterone-booster/ January 4, 2019 (accessed 1/30/19).

Richardson, K., et al. "Anticolinergic Drugs and Risk of Dementia: Case-Control Study." *British Medical Journal*, April 2018.

Risacher, S. L., et al. "Association between Anticholinergic Medication Use and Cognition, Brain Metabolism, and Brain Atrophy in Cognitively Normal Older Adults." *Journal of the American Medical Association–Neurology*, April 2016.

Rohrmann, S., et al. "Serum Estrogen, but Not Testosterone, Levels Differ between Black and White Men in a Nationally Representative Sample of Americans." *Journal of Clinical Endocrinology and Metabolism*, July 2007.

Roy, C. N., et al. "Association of Testosterone Levels with Anemia in Older Men: A Controlled Clinical Trial." *Journal of the American Medical Association–Internal Medicine*, April 2017.

Rubin, D. A., et al. "Endocrine Response to Acute Resistance Exercise in Obese Versus Lean Physically Active Men." *European Journal of Applied Physiology*, June 2015.

Russo, A., et al. "Sereno Repens, Selenium and Lycopene to Manage Lower Urinary Tract Symptoms Suggestive for Benign Prostatic Hyperplasia." *Expert Opinon on Drug Safety*, December 2016.

Saad, F., et al. "Effects of Long-Term Treatment with Testosterone on Weight and Waist Size in 411 Hypogonadal Men with Obesity Classes 1-III: Observational Data from Two Registry Studies." *International Journal of Obesity*, January 2016.

———. "Testosterone as Potential Effective Therapy in Treatment of Obesity in Men with Testosterone Deficiency: A Review." *Current Diabetes Review*, March 2012.

Saeed, S. A., et al. "Exercise, Yoga, and Meditation for Depressive and Anxiety Disorders." *American Family Physician*, April 2010.

Safarineiad, M. R. "Urtica Dioica for Treatment of Benign Prostatic Hyperplasia: A Prospective, Randomized, Double-Blind, Placebo-Controlled, Crossover Study." *Journal of Herbal Pharmacotherapy*, 2005.

Sainj, R. "Coenzyme Q10: The Essential Nutrient." *Journal of Pharmacy and Bioallied Sciences*, July–September 2011.

Samaras, N., et al. "Off-Label Use of Hormones as an Anti-aging Strategy: A Review." *Clinical Interventions in Aging*, 2014.

Schmitt, E. B., et al. "Vitamin D Deficiency Is Associated with Metabolic Syndrome in Postmenopausal Women." *Maturitas*, January 2018.

Schulster, M., et al. "The Role of Estradiol in Male Reproductive Function." *Asian Journal of Andrology*, May–June 2016.

Schulte, D. M., et al. "Caloric Restriction Increases Serum Testosterone Concentrations in Obese Male Subjects by Two Distinct Mechanisms." *Hormone and Metabolic Research*, 2014.

Schwarz, E. R., et al. "Andropause and the Development of Cardiovascular Diseases Presentation—More Than an Epi-phenomenon." *Journal of Geratric Cardiology*, March 2011.

ScienceDaily. "Too Much Sugar Turns Off Gene That Controls Effects of Sex Steroids." November 21, 2007. https://www.sciencedaily.com/releases/2007/11/071109171610.htm.

———. "Testosterone Therapy Does Not Raise Risk of Aggressive Prostate Cancer." May 7, 2016. www.sciencedaily.com/releases/2016/05/160507143326.htm (accessed 3/15/2019).

Scudese, E., et al. "Long Rest Interval Promotes Durable Testosterone Responses in High-Intensity Bench Press." *Journal of Strength and Conditioning Research*, May 2016.

Seidman, S. N. "Normative Hypogonadism and Depression: Does 'Andropause' Exist?" *International Journal of Impotence Research*, 2006.

Shah, G. R., et al. "Evaluation of a Multi-herb Supplement for Erectile Dysfunction: A Randomized Double-Blind, Placebo-Controlled Study." *BMC Complementary and Alternative Medicine*, September 2012.

Shankar, U. S., et al. "Effects of Testosterone on Muscle Strength, Physical Function, Body Composition, and Quality of Life in Intermediate-Frail and Frail Elderly Men: A Randomized, Double-Blind, Placebo-Controlled Study." *Journal of Clinical Endocrinoloy and Metabolism*, February 2010.

Sharma, R., et al. "Normalization of Testosterone Level Is Associated with Reduced Incidence of Myocardial Infarction and Mortality in Men." *European Heart Journal*, October 2015.

———. "Normalization of Testosterone Levels after Testosterone Replacement Therapy Is Associated with Decreased Incidence of Atrial Fibrillation." *Journal of the American Heart Association*, May 2017.

Shell, W., et al. "A Randomized Placebo-Controlled Trial of an Amino Acid Preparation on Timing and Quality of Sleep." *American Journal of Therapeutics*, March–April 2010.

Shenoy, S., et al. "Effects of Eight-Week Supplementation of Ashwagandha on Cardiorespiratory Endurance in Elite Indian Cyclists." *Journal of Ayurveda and Integrated Medicine*, October 2012.

Sher, L. "Both High and Low Testosterone Levels May Play a Role in Suicidal Behavior in Adolescent, Young, Middle-Age, and Older Men: A Hypothesis." *International Journal of Adolescent Medicine and Health*, June 2016.

———. "Low Testosterone Levels May Be Associated with Suicidal Behavior in Older Men while High Testosterone Levels May Be Related to Suicidal Behavior in Adolescents and Young Adults: A Hypothesis." *International Journal of Adolescent Medicine and Health*, 2013.

Shigehara, K., et al. "Effects of Testosterone Replacement Therapy on Hypogonadal Men with Osteopenia or Osteoporosis: A Subanalysis of a Prospective Randomized Controlled Study in Japan." *Aging Male*, September 2017.

Shin, S. S., and M. Yoon. "Korean Red Ginseng (Panax Ginseng) Inhibits Obesity and Improves Lipid Metabolism in High Fat Diet-Fed Castrated Mice." *Journal of Ethnopharmacology*, January 2018.

Shores, M. M., et al. "Increased Incidence of Diagnosed Depressive Illness in Hypogonadal Older Men." *Archives of General Psychiatry*, February 2004.

Shoskes, J. J., et al. "Pharmacology and Testosterone Replacement Therapy Preparations." *Translational Andrology and Urology*, December 2016.

Shukla, K. K., et al. "Mucuna Pruriens Improves Male Fertility by Its Actions on the Hypothalamus-Pituitary-Gonadal Axis." *Fertility and Sterility*, December 2009.

Silva, A. B., et al. "Physical Activity and Exercise for Erectile Dysfunction: Systematic Review and Meta-analysis." *British Journal of Sports Medicine*, October 2017.

Skinner, J. W., et al. "Muscular Responses to Testosterone Replacement Vary by Administration Route: A Systematic Review and Meta-analysis." *Journal of Cachexia Sarcopenia and Muscle*, June 2018.

Snyder, P. J., et al. "Effect of Testosterone Treatment on Volumetric Bone Density and Strength in Older Men with Low Testosterone: A Controlled Clinical Trial." *Journal of the American Medical Association–Internal Medicine*, April 2017.

Sobajima, M., et al. "Waon Therapy Improves Quality of Life as Well as Cardiac Function and Exercise Capacity in Patients with Chronic Heart Failure." *International Heart Journal*, 2015.

Sripada, R. K., et al. "DHEA Enhances Emotion Regulation Neurocircuits Andmodulates Memory for Emotional Stimuli." *Neuropsychopharmacology*, August 2013.

Stanley, T. L., and S. K. Grinspoon. "Effects of Growth Hormone-Releasing Hormone on Visceral Fat, Metabolic, and Cardiovascular Indices in Human Studies." *Growth Hormone and IGF Research*, April 2015.

Steels, E., et al. "Physiological Aspects of Male Libido Enhanced by Standardized Trigonella Foenum-Graecum Extract and Mineral Formulation." *Phytotherapy Research*, September 2011.

Stein, R. A., et al. "*Kaempferia parviflora* Ethanol Extract Improves Self-Assessed Sexual Health in Men: A Pilot Study." *Journal of International Medicine*, July 2018.

Stephenson, J., et al. "Before the Beginning: Nutrition and Lifestyle in the Preconception Period and Its Importance for Future Health." *Lancet*, May 2018.

Stone, N. N., et al. "Male Androgen Deficiency Syndrome Screening Questionnaire: A Simplified Instrument to Identify Testosterone-Deficient Men." *Journal of Men's Health*, April 2014.

Storer, T. W., et al. "Effects of Testosterone Supplementation for 3 Years on Muscle Performance and Physical Function in Older Men." *Journal of Clinical Endocrinology and Metabolism*, February 2017.

Tachikawa, E., and K. Kudo. "Proof of the Mysterious Efficacy of Ginseng: Basic and Clinical Trials: Suppression of Adrenal Medullary Function in Vitro by Ginseng." *Journal of Pharmacological Sciences*, June 2004.

Tacklind, J., et al. "Serenoa Repens for Benign Prostatic Hyperplasia." *Cochrane Database Systematic Review*, December 2012.

Tai, Paul Ling. "For a Younger Tomorrow: Saliva Hormone Testing Is the First Step to Extending Your Youthful Years." *Healing Our World* 38, no. 4, October 2018. www.hippocratesinstituate.org.

Takeda, A., et al. "Recombinant Human Growth Hormone for the Treatment of Growth Disorders in Children: A Systematic Review and Economic Evaluation." *Health Technology Assessment*, September 2010.

Tambi, M., et al. "Standardised Water-Soluble Extract of Eurycoma Longifolia, as Testosterone Booster for Managing Men with Late-Onset Hypogonadism?" *Andrologia*, May 2012.

Tavares, A., et al. "Effects of Growth Hormone Administration on Muscle Strength in Men Over 50 Years Old." *Internationl Journal of Endocrinology*, November 2013.

Thomas, G. A., et al. "Immunoreactive and Bioactive Growth Hormone Responses to Resistance Exercise in Men Who Are Lean or Obese." *Journal of Applied Physiology*, August 2011.

Tirabassi, G., et al. "Vitamin D and Male Sexual Function: A Transversal and Longitudinal Study." *International Journal of Endocrinology*, January 2018.

Tiscione, D., et al. "Daidzein Plus Isolase Associated with Zinc Improves Clinical Symptoms and Quality of Life in Patients with LUTS Due to Benign Prostatic Hyperplasia: Results From a Phase 1-II Study." *Archives Italian Urolology and Andrology*, March 2017.

Toma, M., et al. "Testosterone Supplementation in Heart Failure: A Meta-analysis." *Circulation Heart Failure*, May 2012.

Toogood, A. A., et al. "Beyond the Somatopause: Growth Hormone Deficiency in Adults over the Age of 60 Years." *Journal of Clinical Endocrinology and Metabolism*, 1995.

Traish, A. M. "Testosterone and Weight Loss: The Evidence." *Current Opinion in Endocrinology & Diabetes and Obesity*, October 2014.

Traish, A. M., et al. "Long-Term Testosterone Therapy Improves Cardiometabolic Function and Reduces Risk of Cardiovascular Disease in Men with Hypogonadism: A Real-Life Observational Registry Study Setting Comparing Treated and Untreated (Control) Groups." *Journal of Cardiovascular Pharmacology and Therapeutics*, September 2017.

———. "Long-Term Testosterone Therapy in Hypogonadal Men Ameliorates Elements of the Metabolic Syndrome: An Observational, Long-Term Registry Study." *International Journal of Clinical Practice*, March 2014.

———. "The Dark Side of Testosterone Deficiency: Metabolic Syndrome and Erectile Dysfunction." *Journal of Andrology*, January–February 2009.

———. "The Dark Side of Testosterone Deficiency II: Type 2 Diabetes and Insulin Resistance." *Journal of Andrology*, January–February 2009.

———. "The Dark Side of Testosterone Deficiency III: Cardiovascular Disease." *Journal of Andrology*, September–October 2009.

Trasande, L., et al. "Association of Exposure to Di-2-Ethylhexylphthalate Replacements with Increased Blood Pressure in Children and Adolescents." *Hypertension*, July 2015.

Trauer, J. W., et al. "Cognitive Behavioral Therapy for Chronic Insomnia: A Systematic Review and Meta-analysis." *Annals of Internal Medicine*, 2015.

Travison, T. G., et al. "A Population-Level Decline in Serum Testosterone Levels in American Men." *Journal of Clinical Endocrinology and Metabolism*, January 2007.

Truong, V. L., et al. "Hair Regenerative Mechanisms of Red Ginseng Oil and Its Major Components in the Testosterone-Induced Delay of Anagen Entry in C57BL/6 Mice." *Molecules*, September 2017.

U.S. National Institutes of Health, Office of Dietary Supplements. "Vitamin B12: Fact Sheet for Health Professionals." https://ods.nih.gov/factsheets/vitaminb12-healthprofessional/ (accessed 12/1/18).

U.S. National Library of Medicine. "Androgenetic Alopecia." https://ghr.nlm.nih.gov/condition/androgenetic-alopecia#genes (accessed 11/11/18).

University of California, Davis. "Sleep, Stress and Relaxation." https://shcs.ucdavis.edu/sites/default/files/documents/conquering_insomnia_session-04.pdf (accessed 1/8/19).

University of Iowa Health Care. "Keeping Older Muscles Strong." September 8, 2015.

Vahlensieck, W., et al. "Effects of Pumpkin Seed in Men with Lower Urinary Tract Symptoms Due to Benign Prostatic Hyperplasia in the One-Year, Randomized, Placebo-Controlled GRANU Study." *Urology International*, 2015.

Van Heukelom, R. O., et al. "Influence of Melatonin on Fatigue Severity in Patients with Chronic Fatigue Syndrome and Late Melatonin Secretion." *European Journal of Neurology*, January 2006.

Varshavsky, J. R., et al. "Dietary Sources of Cumulative Phthalates Exposure among the U.S. General Population in NHANES 2005–2014." *Environment International*, June 2018.

Velazquez, M. A., T. Fleming, and A. J. Watkins. "Periconceptual Environment and the Developmental Origins of Disease." *Journal of Endocrinology*, February 2019.

Vinarov, A. Z., et al. "Effect of Transdermal Testosterone on the Quality of Life of Men with Androgen Deficiency and Chronic Prostatitis in Routine Clinical Practice." *Urologia*, March 2018.

Wahjoepramono, E. J., et al. "The Effects of Testosterone Supplementation on Cognitive Functioning in Older Men." *CNS and Neurological Disorders Drug Targets*, 2016.

Wallace, M. B., et al. "Effects of Dehydroepiandrosterone vs. Androstenedione Supplementation in Men." *Medicine and Science in Sports and Exercise*, December 1999.

Walsh, T. J., et al. "Testosterone Treatment and the Risk of Aggressive Prostate Cancer in Men with Low Testosterone Levels." *PLOS One*, June 2018.

Wang, F., et al. "Erectile Dysfunction and Fruit/Vegetable Consumption among Diabetic Canadian Men." *Urology*, December 2013.

Wang, W., et al. "Cigarette Smoking Has a Positive and Independent Effect on Testosterone Levels." *Hormones*, October–December 2013.

Watanabe, K., et al. "Marijuana Extracts Possess the Effects Like the Endocrine Disrupting Chemicals." *Toxicology*, January 2005.

WebMD. "Off-Label Drug Use: What You Need to Know." https://www.webmd.com/a-to-z-guides/features/off-label-drug-use-what-you-need-to-know#1 (accessed 2/1/19).

Witorsch, R. J., et al. "Personal Care Products and Endocrine Disruption: A Critical Review of the Literature." *Critical Reviews in Toxicology*, November 2010.

Wong, T. H., et al. "Effects of 25-Hydroxyvitamin D and Vitamin D-Binding Protein on Bone Mineral Density and Disease Activity in

Malaysian Patients with Rheumatoid Arthritis." *International Journal of Rheumatic Diseases*, May 2018.

Wu, A., et al. "Curcumin Boosts DHA in the Brain: Implications for the Prevention of Anxiety Disorders." *Biochimica et Biophysica Acta*, May 2015.

Xie, Z., et al. "A Review of Sleep Disorders and Melatonin." *Neurological Research*, June 2017.

Yang, O., et al. "Endocrine-Disrupting Chemicals: Review of Toxicological Mechanisms Using Molecular Pathway Analysis." *Journal of Cancer Prevention*, March 2015.

Yassin, D. J., et al. "Long-Term Testosterone Treatment in Elderly Men with Hypogonadism and Erectile Dysfunction Reduces Obesity Parameters and Improves Metabolic Syndrome and Health-Related Quality of Life." *Journal of Sexual Medicine*, June 2014.

Ye, L., et al. "Dietary Patterns and Depression Risk: A Meta-analysis." *Psychiatry Research*, July 2017.

Yeap, B. B., et al. "In Older Men, Higher Plasma Testosterone or Dihydrotestosterone Is an Independent Predictor for Reduced Incidence of Stroke but Not Myocardial Infarction." *Journal of Clinical Endocrinology and Metabolism*, December 2014.

Yimam, M., et al. "A Botanical Composition Mitigates Cartilage Degradations and Pain Sensitivity in Osteoarthritis Disease Model." *Journal of Medicinal Food*, June 2017.

———. "UP1306, a Botanical Compositions with Analgesic and Anti-Inflammatory Effect." *Pharmacognosy Research*, July–September 2016.

Zhang, J., et al. "Both Total Testosterone and Sex Hormone–Binding Globulin Are Independent Risk Factors for Metabolic Syndrome: Results from Fangchenggang Area Male Health and Examination Survey in China." *Diabetes/Metabolism Research and Reviews*, July 2013.

Zhang, N. N., et al. "Hair Growth–Promoting Activity of Hot Water Extract of Thuja Orientalis." *BMC Complementary and Alternative Medicine*, January 2013.

Zhanzhan, L., et al. "Growth Hormone Replacement Therapy Reduces Risk of Cancer in Adult with Growth Hormone Deficiency: A Meta-analysis." *Oncotarget*, December 2016.

Zhu, W., et al. "A Review of Traditional Pharmacological Uses, Phytochemistry, and Pharmacological Activities of *Tribulus terrestris*." *Chemistry Central Journal*, 2017.

Zota, A. R., et al. "Recent Fast Food Consumption and Bisphenol A and Phtyalates Exposures among the U.S. Population in NHANES, 2003–2010." *Environmental Health Perspectives*, October 2016.

Index

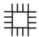

dihomo-y-linolenicacid (DGLA), 69
dihydrotestosterone (DHT), 14, 65–67
diseases, 25–27, 29–30, 37, 39–40. *See also specific diseases*
doping, 156–57
drugs. *See* pharmaceutical drugs
Duke University, 37–38
dutasteride, 67

early-onset andropause, 25
Eclipta alba, 68
ED. *See* erectile dysfunction
Endocrine Disrupting Chemicals, 97
endocrines, 96–97
Environmental Toxicology, 34
Environmental Working Group, 33
Epstein, Samuel S., 32
erectile dysfunction (ED), 92;
    aging and, 171; with IMS, 169;
    metabolism and, 116; natural
    solutions for, 119–27; research
    on, 118–19, 123, 126–27;
    shockwave treatment for, 117.
    See also sexual dysfunction
estradiol, 22–23, 92
estrogen, 13, 91, 138, 155
ethnicity, 22–23, 35, 40–41, 108
Eurycoma longifolia. *See* Malaysian ginseng
exercise: aerobic, 160–61; cognitive
    decline and, 42–43; CVD and,
    143; diet and, 6; fatigue and,
    72–73; for insomnia, 87–88;
    intervention, 117–18; against
    obesity, 97; vigorous, 160–61

far-infrared saunas, 38
fast food, 35–37

fatigue, 9; chronic, 38, 71–77; from
    diabetes, 103; exercise and, 72–
    73; natural solutions for, 73–76;
    TRT for, 76–77
fat mass, 62
FDA. *See* Food and Drug Administration
fenugreek (*Trigonella foenum-graecum*), 73, 124
fiber, 100
finasteride, 67
Fitzgerald, Randall, 15, 131
flame retardants, 37–38
Food and Drug Administration
    (FDA), 133–35, 140, 156
Forsythe, James, 162–63
frailty, 59, 76–77, 158
free hormones, 139–40
Frontiers of Nutrition, 44
full-spectrum liquid ginseng, 166
Furosap, 124

Gabadone, 86
gastric bypass surgery, 98
gender failure, 3–4
George Washington University, 35–36
GH. *See* growth hormone
ginger. *See* Thai black ginger
ginkgo biloba, 66
ginseng: full-spectrum liquid, 166;
    Korean, 80, 101–2, 122–23;
    Malaysian, 122; red ginseng oil,
    67–68; Siberian, 73
glucose. *See* sugar
grapefruit, 30
green drinks, 129–30
green tomatoes, 61
growth hormone (GH): cancer
    and, 157–58; DHEA and, 24;

About the Authors

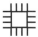

Brian R. Clement, PhD, LN, and his wife, **Anna Maria Clement**, PhD, LN, have spearheaded the international progressive health movement for more than four decades as directors of the renowned Hippocrates Health Institute, in West Palm Beach, Florida, the world's foremost complementary residential health center, which has served more than a half-million clients since its founding. *Spa Magazine* calls Hippocrates "the number one wellness spa in the world."

Over the last half century, this couple and their team of health care professionals have pioneered clinical research and training in disease prevention using hundreds of thousands of participants who provided volumes of data, giving the Clements a privileged insight into the lifestyle required to prevent disease, enhance longevity, and maintain vitality. Their findings have provided the basis for Hippocrates's progressive, state-of-the-art treatments and programs for health maintenance and recovery—their Life Transformation Program.

In addition to their research studies, the Clements conduct dozens of conferences before tens of thousands of people worldwide each year, educating on how to attain health and longevity, and giving humanity a roadmap for enriching their lives.

Individually and together they have authored more than twenty books, including *Living Foods for Optimum Health* (1998); *Hippocrates*

LifeForce (2007), which Cornell University nutritional biochemist Dr. T. Colin Campbell called, in his preface to it, "One of the most important books ever written on nutrition"; *Supplements Exposed* (2009); and *7 Keys to Lifelong Sexual Vitality* (2012).